Remembered Remed
Traditional Scottish P

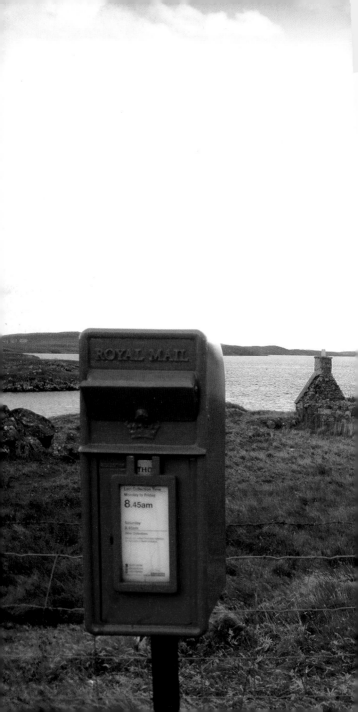

BIRLINN

Remembered Remedies
Traditional Scottish Plant Lore

ANNE BARKER

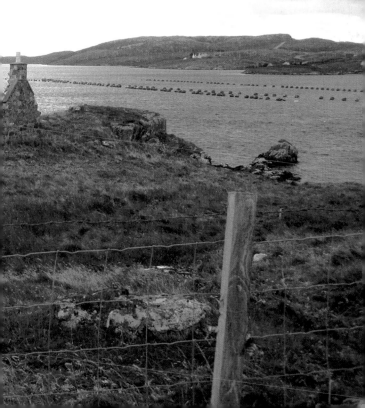

Previous page.
The croft house on the Isle of Great Bernera, Lewis,
where Agnus Maclennan's mother was born

First published in 2011 by
Birlinn Limited
West Newington House
10 Newington Road
Edinburgh
EH9 1QS

www.birlinn.co.uk

ISBN: 978 1 78027 004 3

British Library Cataloguing-in-Publication Data
A catalogue record for this book is available from the British Library

Designed and typeset by Mark Blackadder

Much of the content of this book arises from research conducted for
the Ethnomedica Remembered Remedies project, sponsored in part by
the Royal Botanic Gardens, Kew, where the project's archive is held;
material from that archive is used by kind permission of Ethnomedica
Remembered Remedies and the Royal Botanic Gardens, Kew.

Printed in Europe on behalf of Latitute Press Ltd

℘ Contents

❦ Vegetables and kitchen cures

ও Acknowledgements

I am grateful to the Royal Botanic Gardens, Kew, which, through the Ethnomedica project, provided funding for collecting trips to the Isles of Skye and Mull, to Sutherland and Easter Ross, and to St Andrews in 2007, 2008 and 2009. Mary Beith, a tremendous inspiration, has provided me with some of her own memories of plant uses, and those that had been told to her in days gone by. Lynn Goodlad at the Shetland Library located the reference to the local Yell name for a plant.

David Chamberlain helped with mosses. Gabrielle Hatfield read the manuscript and gave helpful suggestions. Greg Kenicer advised on recent changes in taxonomy. Thanks to Richard Milne and Heather McHaffie for contributing their photographs, which are noted in the text. All other photographs are mine. Thanks also to the many contributors who helped me with my research over the past four years, including those living in St Andrews, Easter Ross, Sutherland, Skye, Mull, Argyll, Orkney, Lewis and the Shetlands.

Anne Barker MNIMH
Ethnomedica Scotland Co-ordinator

❧ *Foreword*

For at least 300 years, many collectors of the traditional remedies and other plant uses of Scotland have regreted that their researches hadn't begun 20, 40, or 50 years earlier. So much knowledge appeared to have been lost, yet the ploughing of the old ground continues to turn up fresh treasures of local ingenuity.

Anne Barker, who brings an expert herbalist's understanding to country traditions, has dug out much fascinating oral information which lends new aspects to old practices and, indeed, several hitherto unrecorded uses. *Remembered Remedies* is a welcome addition to a captivating subject and has something to surprise and delight even the most dedicated follower of plant lore.

Mary Beith
May 2011

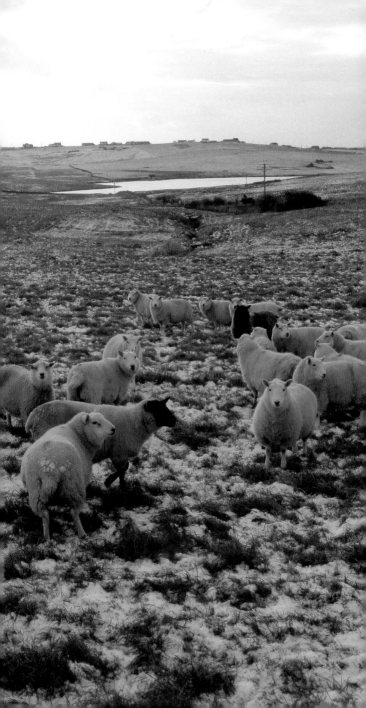

֎ Disclaimer

This book contains information on both edible and medicinal plants. Some of these medicinal uses have not been tested in recent times and cannot be guaranteed to be safe. If medicinal or edible plants are misidentified or misused, there is a danger of poisoning. Therefore it is not recommended that you try the edible species unless you are confident that you can identify them correctly. It is also recommended that you do not experiment with medicinal uses, especially internal ones, without seeking further advice, including accurate dosage instructions, from a qualified medical herbalist.

Some British plant species are protected by law and must not be picked in the wild. It is also illegal to uproot any plant on private land without the owner's permission or to pick plants in officially protected areas. The author cannot accept any responsibility for any medical problems suffered by readers as a consequence of experimenting with plants, nor for any breaches of the Wildlife and Countryside Act 1987 or subsequent revisions of that Act.

Opposite.
Sheep on the croft, Skelberry, Dunrossness, Shetland, November 2010

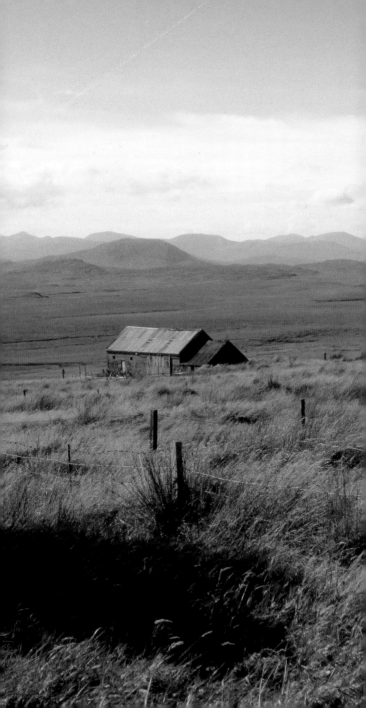

✌ *Introduction*

The oral tradition of plant folklore, where knowledge is passed on by word of mouth rather than the printed page, is important because it represents a repository of actual plant use as well as the understanding of the significance of plants in our culture. Over the past four years, I have been collecting the plant stories in this book for the Ethnomedica project. All the raw material I have collected has been added to the project's archive at the Royal Botanic Gardens, Kew. This book is my record of those collections. In travelling about Scotland, I have listened to people's memories of using simple remedies: gathering hips, haws and the red moss during the two World Wars, collecting seaweed from island shores, using garden vegetables, bottling cordials, making heather beds and chaff mattresses during harvest time, and making do with what was to hand when the doctor was many miles away and there was no money to pay for his visit. It was clear to me that many of these plant uses had been handed down over several generations. In this book, I have organised the stories I collected by general habitat (seashore, meadow, hedgerow, etc.) and further

Opposite.
Byre, Achmore, Lewis, September 2010

by plant name. I have added botanical information about plant habitat and distribution, and there is a table of plant classification at the end of the book.

Over the past four hundred years in Scotland, a number of collectors have worked in this field. The first recorded collections of traditional plant uses, in the late 17th and early 18th centuries, were those of Martin Martin, a Gaelic-speaking native of Skye. He was sent by the Royal Society to visit the Isles of Lewis and St Kilda, and his accounts of the journey included local plant lore, in which he was very interested. In 1772, the botanist John Lightfoot toured Scotland and produced the *Flora Scotica,* classifying plants by the new Linnaean taxonomy, but also including Gaelic plant names and traditional uses of plants. At about the same time (1767–71), James Robertson was commissioned by the Royal Botanic Garden, Edinburgh to record natural history in Scotland; he too included traditional plant uses together with his lists of flora and fauna. William MacGillivray, who had spent his childhood in the Hebrides, wrote about traditional Hebridean plant uses in 1831. But by the second half of the 19th century knowledge of plant folklore was disappearing in Scotland. The linguistic scholar John Cameron, in his *Gaelic Names of Plants* (1883), attempted to remedy the absence of any compendium of Gaelic plant names. Murdoch McNeill in his flora *Colonsay* (1910) included Gaelic plant names as well as traditional plant uses.[1]

Alexander Carmichael, a native Gaelic speaker from Lismore, travelled about the Highlands and Islands as an excise man, and collected oral Gaelic traditions throughout the second half of the 19th century; these were published at the beginning of the 20th century.[2] Iain F. Campbell (John Francis Campbell) of Islay, a scholar of Gaelic folk literature, published some of Carmichael's early work; he accompanied Carmichael on a collecting trip to South Uist in 1871.[3] Plant uses were often embedded in the oral Gaelic folklore Carmichael recorded: for example, charms about yarrow, St John's Wort and Mòthan.[4]

More recently, Mary Beith[5] wrote about traditional remedies of the Highlands and Islands from the standpoint of social history. In this century, botanists William Milliken and Sam Bridgewater researched the uses of plants in Scotland in the past and present. Having interviewed members of the public for the Flora Celtica archive, they observed that little of the oral traditional plant lore remains alive today in Scotland[6]; however, my experience in collecting for Ethnomedica in Scotland would suggest otherwise.

Nevertheless, the oral tradition of folk knowledge about our plants in Britain is in danger of dying out and needs to be preserved. For this reason, Ethnomedica, known as 'Remembered Remedies', was set up more than ten years ago as an oral history project by medical herbalists and ethnobotanists in Britain. The project aims to record and research traditional medical British plant lore, particularly from the period before the National Health Service came into being in 1947, thus preserving the wealth of knowledge about local uses of plants as medicines. The information gathered by Ethnomedica volunteer collectors is added to the project's archive and database at the Royal Botanic Gardens, Kew. Collectors for the project record the uses

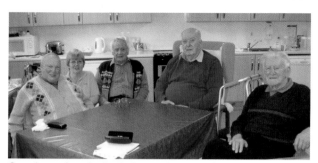

Contributors from Sandwick, Cunningsburgh and Quarff at Overton Lea Day Centre, Levenwick, Shetland, November 2010

of plants and their associated stories from the oral testimony of contributors throughout Britain. By the end of 2009, more than 5,000 remedies had been recorded, including more than four hundred and fifty different plant species.

Ethnomedica is a collaborative, non-profit organisation supported by the National Institute of Medical Herbalists; the Royal Botanic Gardens, Kew; Chelsea Physic Garden; the Eden Project; the Natural History Museum and the Royal Botanic Garden, Edinburgh. Contributors may write directly to the project to offer their 'Remembered Remedies' for inclusion in the archive:

Ethnomedica – Remembered Remedies
Royal Botanic Gardens, Kew
Richmond, Surrey TW9 3AB
email: ethnomedica@kew.org

Field, meadow and machair

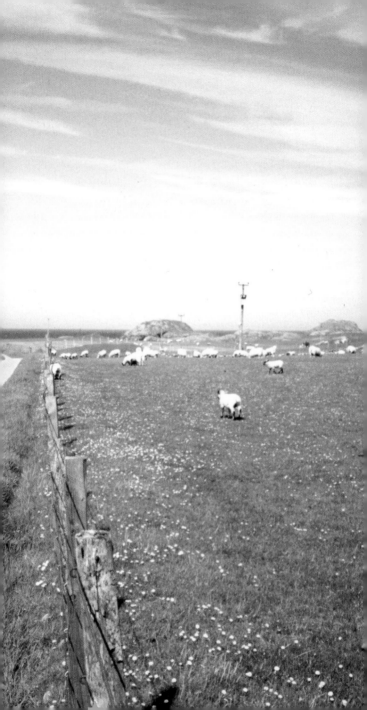

℘ *Betony*

A man from the Isle of Raasay related that what he called 'Bethony', a plant with blue flowers, was collected, dried and taken as tea there. He said the tea was 'very pleasant-tasting'. Interestingly enough, although he is a Gaelic speaker, he didn't use a Gaelic name for the plant.

Wood betony (*Stachys officinalis*) flowers from June to October, and grows in grassy places and heaths, avoiding clay, and preferring limestone; it is common in England and Wales, and can be found locally in lowland Scotland, but most floras indicate that wood betony is generally absent from the north of Scotland and the Isles.[7] Morag Henriksen[8] told me subsequently that it had been recorded on Raasay, as well as around the ruins of a tower above the pier in Portree where a monastic dwelling is thought to have been.

Opposite. Iona, towards the Machair
Below. Betony (Richard Milne)

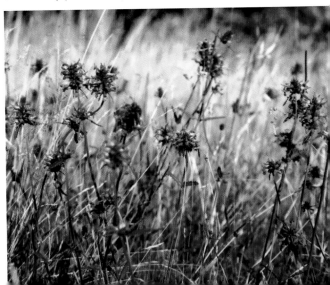

𝒫𝒶 *Butterwort and Milkwort*

A woman from Balmaqueen, Skye, said that there were two flowers associated with cows. The cows were not happy unless they got the *blue* one (see below) for the milk (thyme-leaved milkwort, *Polygala serpyllifolia*, Gaelic 'Siabann nam Ban-sìdh', meaning 'Fairy Women's Soap'[9]) and the *yellow* one (right) for the colour of the butter (common butterwort, *Pinguicula vulgaris*, Gaelic 'Mòthan', meaning 'Bog Violet'[10]).

Butterwort flowers from May to July on wet rocks, bogs and wet heaths throughout most of Scotland, particularly the Highlands, the Northern Isles and the Hebrides. It is common in Wales, Northern Ireland and

Milkwort (Heather McHaffie)

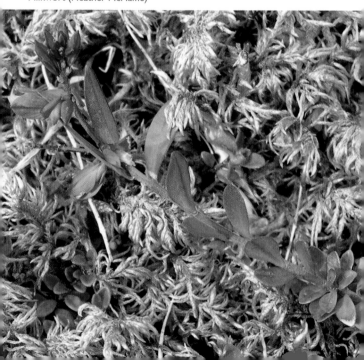

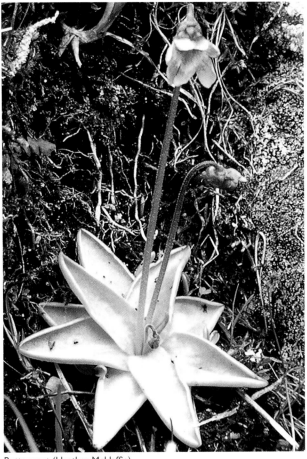

Butterwort (Heather McHaffie)

northern England but relatively absent in the south of England.[11] The thyme-leaved milkwort, flowering from March to October, is widely distributed in Britain, especially in the north-west Highlands and Islands, Orkney and Shetland, on dry, lime-free, acid heaths and grassland.[12]

৯৯ *Chaff*

A man in Skinnet, Sutherland, said that the old women loved their chaff mattresses. When, in pre-war Talmine, the grain (oats, *Avena sativa*) was being winnowed, 'the old women would come down from the hills' and collect the chaff into sacks, which were then used as mattresses. They refilled or replaced the chaff each year. The chaff mattresses were then put over the top of the heather beds (Heather, p.57). A man from Altandubh, Wester Ross, remembers that before the First World War his mother originally had chaff mattresses, but he says that they rustled a lot and weren't very comfortable.

Below, a wooden threshing machine from 1929 is at

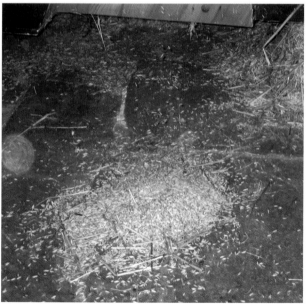

Chaff

work in a barn in Skelberry, Shetland, with the oat chaff top right and the oat grains, centre, emerging from the brown hopper.

A woman from Arbroath in Angus remembers her mother talking about 'caff' mattresses, which she used to sleep on before the Second World War. Her mother came from the Angus countryside and always helped with the harvest, when the mattresses would be filled with new chaff from the winnowed grain. Two women from Birsay, Orkney, both in their eighties, remember chaff, from the threshing of oats, being used for filling mattresses; they thought it was 'lovely when new and cosy'.

🌿 Eyebright

Hazel Gray in Camb, Mid Yell, Shetland, told me that in 1980 she was told by a woman in Seafield, Camb, called Ina (who was born in 1920), that when she was a girl of eight, her little sister had persistently sticky eyes. An old woman in the village called Jean (then in her eighties) 'had seen the bairn, and the child's mother said, "It's been like that for weeks and deil da thing[13] will shift it." So Jean said, "Come doon ta me and I'll fix it." Jean gathered up eyebright plants (roots and all), boiled it up, strained it, and made the lass drink it. She put a drop of sugar in the water to be sure she would drink it all. Within a week the sticky eyes were clear.' Jean was born around 1850 in Seafield. Hazel says there are still some clumps of eyebright growing today in the village but that it is not common.

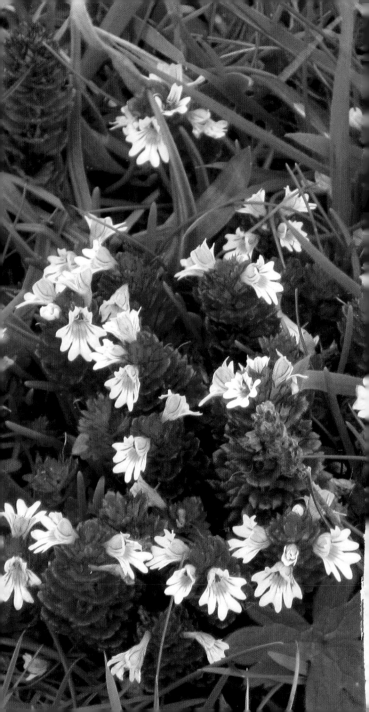

Eyebright (*Euphrasia officinalis*), a partial parasite of grassland, is notoriously difficult to identify, due to species variability and adaptation to local exposure and environment; also there are numerous hybrids, and the species groups have more recently been reclassified.[14] My guess is that in Yell the most likely species of eyebright might be *Euphrasia arctica*,[15] a common native, found in damp meadows and flowering from late May to July. In Gaelic, the plant is known as 'Lus nan Leac', meaning 'Plant of the Hillsides'.[16]

𝓎𝓪 Field Scabious

Around Staffin in Skye, the field scabious (*Knautia arvensis*) is known in Gaelic as 'Gille-Mac-Guirmen[17]': literally, 'The Little Blue Lad'). A small lilac-blue-flowered plant, it has slender stems with button-like heads. A man from Staffin and a woman from nearby Balmaqueen recalled that the flower was used 'for making linen a brighter white'. He added that 'it could also be used as a cure for sores', but 'it's not so plentiful here now as it used to be'. The field scabious flowers from July to September, and grows in dry pastures, grassy fields and banks throughout Britain, although it is less commonly found in the north, and is absent in the Shetlands and Outer Hebrides.[18]

Opposite. Eyebright [19]

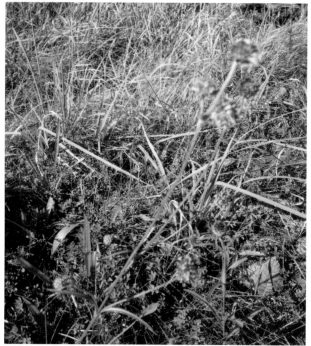

Field Scabious

৯৯ *Foxglove*

According to a man from Staffin, foxgloves (*Digitalis purpurea*) were known there as 'Caileach na mharbh', 'The Thimble of the Dead Lady', as well as 'Old Wives' Thimble'.[20] 'You don't see so many white ones,' said a woman from Balmaqueen. When they were little, these two agreed, they were told not to put foxglove flowers in their mouths.

Opposite. Foxglove (Richard Milne)

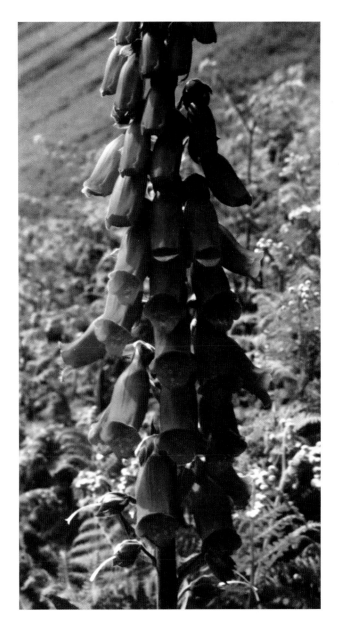

During the Second World War, a friend of mine, then a boy of eleven, was on holiday with his family, staying near Huntly, Aberdeenshire. The chatelaine of the castle nearby organised all the children in the neighbourhood, including the boy and his younger sister, to go out and collect foxglove flowers 'for medicine for the war effort'.

Foxgloves, flowering from June to September, grow on heaths, woodland clearings and burnt moorland in acid soil up to 880 metres throughout most of Britain.[21]

🙢 Meadowsweet

Meadowsweet (*Filipendula ulmaria*), in Gaelic 'Cneas Chù Chulainn' – 'Waist belt of Cuchullin'[22] – is associated with the hero of legend. A woman in Uig on Skye remembered her Lewis grandmother telling her that when Chùchulainn, or Cuchullin, was suffering from shingles, he wrapped the plant around his waist to heal the sores.

Mary Beith spoke of the legendary Cuchullin's terrible temper and how the plant was said to have calmed him down. A woman in Sutherland told me that she would gather the flowers and bring them into the house, putting them in a vase, where the fragrance would cure her terrible headaches. A man from the Isle of Raasay said that the plant was used there for healing. A woman from Balmaqueen on Skye added that it was also used in wine.

Opposite. Meadowsweet (Heather McHaffie)

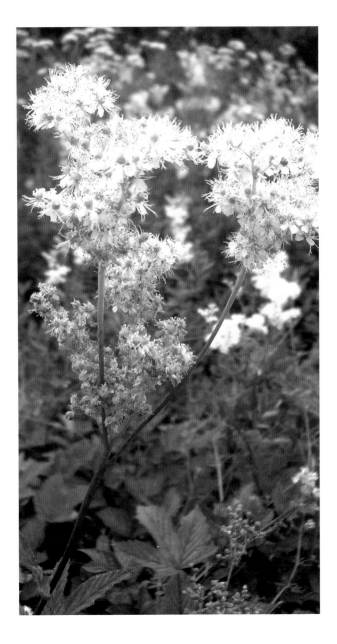

Meadowsweet, flowering from June to September, is found throughout Scotland and the British Isles in fens, marshes, wet woods and meadows, by rivers, and on wet rock ledges up to 915 metres, although it does not grow on very acid peat.[23]

🐟 Oat Straw

In Shetland, a number of croft houses, corn kilns and watermills are still thatched with oat straw (*Avena sativa*).

Bertie Johnson grows oats on his croft, which has been in his family since 1864, at Skelberry, Dunrossness, and supplies oat straw for roofing crofts and watermills to the Shetland Amenity Trust and the Shetland Council. At first he tried growing 'Black Oats', but he remarked

Oat straw-thatched roof near Boddam, Dunrossness, Shetland

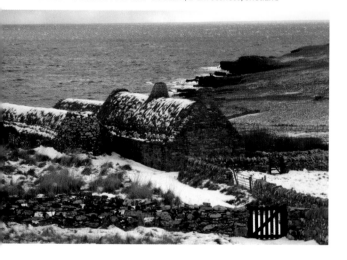

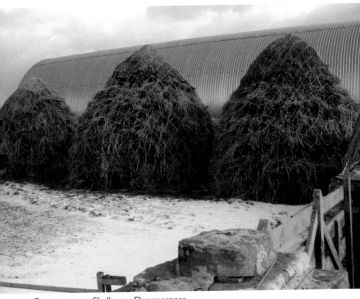

Coarn screws, Skelberry, Dunrossness

that they were 'hellery[24]': they were too floppy and the wind blew them flat in the field so that they couldn't be cut and bound into sheaves. For several years after, he grew the Irish 'Dula' variety, sowing one and a half acres with three hundredweight of seed. However, the Irish straw was too short, and he continued to look for a longer variety. He then tried 'Ayr Bounty', but it was no good for growing in Shetland. Finally, he tried a Finnish variety[25] of oats with a 'hundred day' growing season, and now he is happy. After lambing has finished on the croft in mid-May, he sows the seed in the field where the sheep have been, and harvests the oats in mid-September. The straw is a good three feet tall, and the grain can also be used for grinding into meal (for

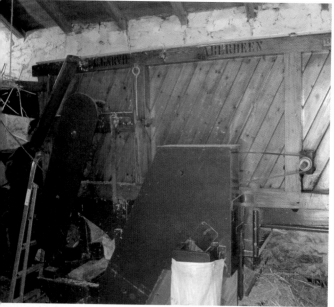

Above. Threshing
Opposite. Trimmed oat straw

people), as well as being fed to sheep, cattle and poultry. He cuts the oats with a binder and makes sheaves a yard high and ten inches in diameter, which are then tied. Ten of these sheaves are gathered together to form a 'stook'; the stooks, in straight strips in the field, are left out for maybe a week. Then he begins to build stacks (a 'dus') from the stooks, starting from the centre, about seven to eight foot in diameter, and pointed at the top, containing about eighty sheaves. The dus stands there in the field until 'cured', another two or three weeks. Then he builds a bigger stack, called a 'screw' (previous page), consisting of about four hundred sheaves.

This is the winter store, and is known in Shetland as

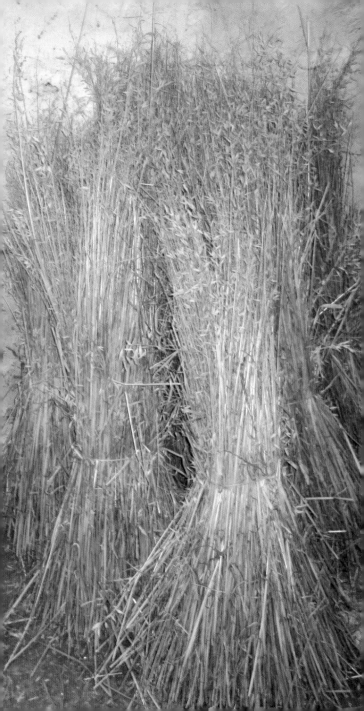

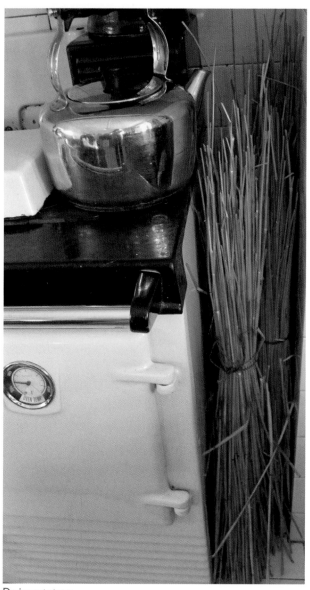

Drying oat straw

'getting the coarn in'. The screw is tied down as follows: Bertie makes a loop of twine at the bottom of the screw, knotting it round a sheaf; then he loops the twine over the top of the screw, around the top once, and then back down to the base of the screw a foot or so along the bottom from the knotted sheaf; after looping the twine round the screw in this way, until it is secured right round, he then finishes by fastening it at the top. When the screw is ready to go into the barn in November, it is unpacked, and the cured sheaves are laid flat in the barn.

Threshing, when the sheaves have their heads cut off, takes place in the barn (p.16); the straw is then bound, trimmed, and stacked vertically (p.17).

One user of Bertie's straw is the Shetland basket-maker Jimmy Work (born in 1924), of Scousburgh, Dunrossness. Jimmy's elder brother Laurie learned how to make oat straw baskets from his father-in-law, 'old Henry Sinclair' (born around 1878). Henry, in turn, had learned how to make them in the Boy Scouts in the early

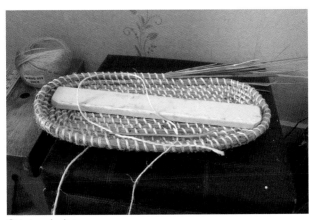

Oat straw basket

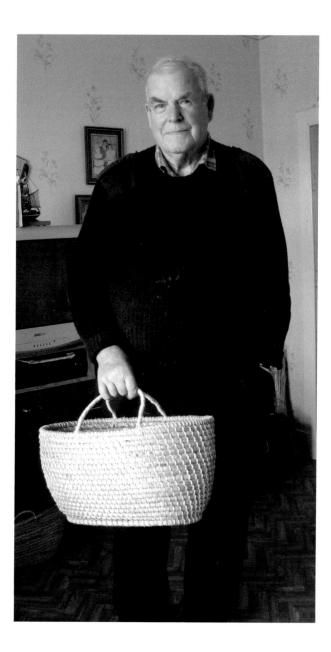

1930s, when he was in his fifties. According to Jimmy, the Boy Scouts ran in Shetland in the 1930s up until the Second World War (then, said Bertie, the Boys' Brigade took hold). Jimmy took up basket-making in 1958, after watching his brother make them. He then decided to improve on his brother's model.

Bertie brings him the prepared sheaves, which Jimmy cures further by stacking them next to his stove for three or four days to be sure the straw is dry – otherwise the baskets will be too floppy. Once dry, he uses oat straw and twine to weave the basket.

He keeps the same number of stitches all the way up the basket, but widens it as he goes (unlike his brother and 'old Henry', who added stitches as the basket widened on the way up). Note how the stitches align on the diagonal in the basket Jimmy is holding.

Pignut

A woman from Balmaqueen, Skye, remembered that 'Braoan' or 'Fairy Hill Bulb' (*Conopodium majus*, pignut;[26] also 'Cnò-thalmhainn', 'Braonan-bhuachaille'[27]) grows on 'wee hills in dry, dry ground', and 'was loved by *very* little pigs'. It had a dark brown covering, she said, which you peeled off, and then ate the 'nut'. Sometimes a beetle would get into the nut. Her friend from Staffin also remembers eating these as a wee boy.

A woman from Bunessan on the Ross of Mull said that 'Lady nuts' grew up with the bracken. You had to be

Opposite. Jimmy Work

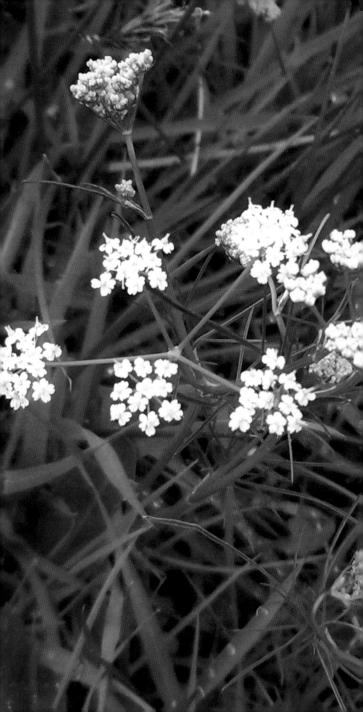

careful to avoid the bracken roots when digging up the 'nuts'. Sometimes, she said, they were double. You scraped off the brown skin and then ate them. She said they tasted like a hazelnut. A woman from Fife said that 'Lucy Arnotts' (a local name for pignut, a Scots dialect corruption of 'lousy earthnuts') were to be found in Kelty Woods during the Second World War.

Pignut, flowering in May and June, is widely found throughout the British Isles in woods and fields, open scrub, grassland and on acid soils; it may possibly have been introduced in the Western Isles.[28]

℘ Silverweed

Silverweed (*Potentilla anserina*) is known in Gaelic as 'Brisghean' or 'Brisgean' ('Brittle One'[29]). A man in Staffin

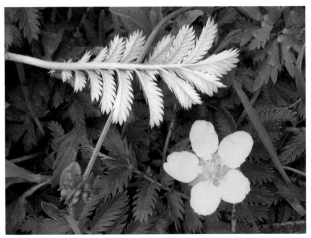

Opposite. Pignut (Heather McHaffie)
Above. Silverweed (Heather McHaffie)

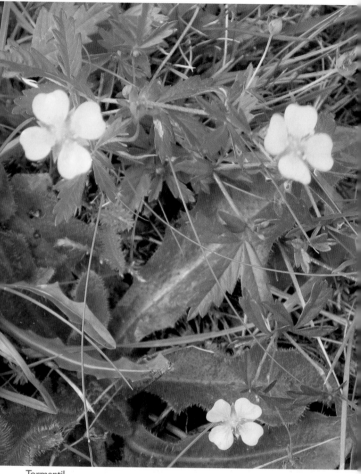

Tormentil

told me that there is a place nearby called 'Lach na Brisghean' – the 'Hollow of the Brittle One', referring to the silverweed that grows round about it. He said that when you put the silverweed in water, it was like silver coins (the water droplets collecting on the leaves). The root is edible, and as children they dug up the roots and ate them. He had heard that in the past the roots were ground up and made into a kind of pudding. Mòr Macleod remembered that as a child in the early 1920s in Earshader, Lewis, in April, she would dig up the root – it was white – of 'Brisghean', wash it and eat it raw. Or she would roast the root over the peat ashes and embers of the open fire in the house. She said that the cattle were very fond of it.

A woman in Bunessan on the Ross of Mull recalled that tormentil (*Potentilla erecta*, left, related to silverweed) was called 'Sheep's nappity' when she was a child. A woman in Dounby, Orkney, said that in 1930, on the Isle of Rousay, she and her older cousin Margaret used to wander up the hill every Sunday. Margaret pointed out the wee yellow flower of tormentil growing among the heather and said that it was good for diarrhoea. The woman heard that it did work, but wasn't sure how it was prepared, although it would 'likely be the root'. Jill Blackadder of Scalloway, Shetland, told me that in the mid-1980s she was told by a local Olaberry man that in the 1920s and '30s he and his siblings were encouraged to dig up and chew the fresh roots of the 'Bark Flooer'[30] to quell hunger pangs, especially before the evening meal.

Silverweed flowers in summer, and is found up to 430 metres all over Scotland and throughout the British Isles, including Orkney and Shetland, in damp grassland or pastures, roadsides and sand dunes, where it can be dominant. Tormentil also flowers in summer, and can be found throughout Britain on moors, heaths, mountainsides, bogs and scrub, where it prefers acid soil.[31]

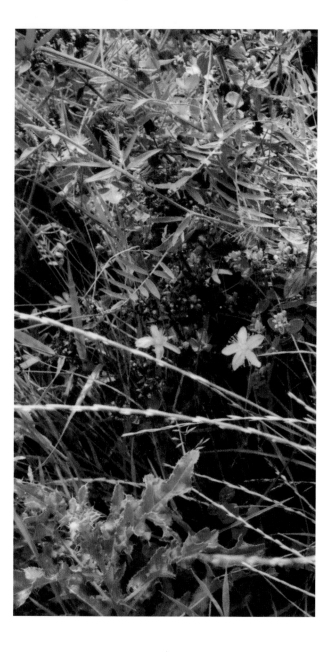

❦ St John's Wort

A man from the Isle of Raasay told me that St John's Wort (*Hypericum pulchrum*, the Slender St John's Wort, Gaelic 'Lus Chaluim chille', 'St Columba's Plant'[32]) was used directly on a cut as a wound herb to prevent infections. Mary Beith reports a similar usage from the Highlands.[33]

The perforate St John's Wort (*H. perforatum*), known as 'Beachnuadh Boireann'[34] in Gaelic, is found especially on chalky soils in woods, hedgebanks and grasslands in the south of Scotland, England and Wales, but is absent from the north-west Highlands, parts of Caithness, the Hebrides and the Northern Isles. Conversely, the slender version (*H. pulchrum*) prefers acid soils in heathy and grassy places, where it is the most common version in the north and west of Scotland, the Northern Isles and the Hebrides.[35]

❦ Yarrow

In Staffin on the Isle of Skye, Yarrow (*Achillea millefolium*), called 'Lus na fala' in Skye Gaelic, was known as a wound herb used to stop bleeding. According to Scott,[36] another Gaelic name for yarrow is 'Eàrr-thalmainn' or 'Tail of the Earth'. If you look at the leaves, they resemble a tail.

A woman from nearby Balmaqueen said that her mother had shown her how to prepare it: you gently boil

Opposite. St John's Wort

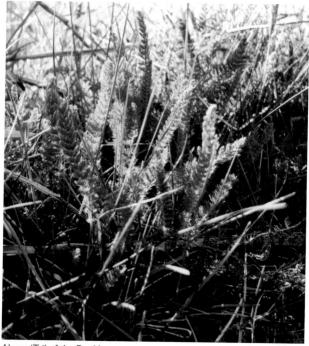

Above. 'Tail of the Earth'
Opposite. Yarrow

it (every bit of the plant – roots, leaves, stems, flowers),
let it cool, strain it and put it on the affected part as a
poultice. She has lots of it growing about her house,
which is at the top of the island.

Grazing animals avoid the strongly bitter-tasting
leaves; hence it is found more abundantly in grazed
pastures throughout Scotland, including the Northern
Isles and the Hebrides. Yarrow flowers in summer,
where, except on the poorest soils, it is commonly found
throughout Britain in meadows, hedgerows, waysides
and grassy banks.[37]

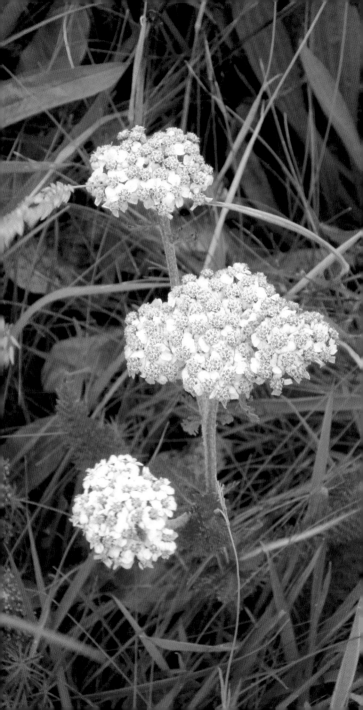

𝔰𝔞 *Yellow Rattle*

Both Hazel Gray, who grew up at Aywick, Mid Yell, Shetland, in the early 1960s, and Helen Jamieson, whose childhood began before the First World War in Gossabrough, East Yell, remember gathering 'Dog's Pennies', the local name[38] for yellow rattle (*Rhinanthus minor*), to use as 'play' money. Helen remembers that the dog's pennies were the size of an old silver thrupenny bit. A Shetland native, the yellow rattle (a partial parasite of grassland) is commonly found in wet and dry meadows, verges and stony heath throughout Scotland and the rest of Britain, and flowers from May to September.[39]

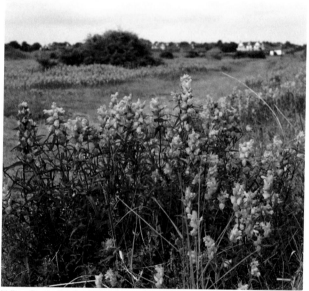

Yellow Rattle (Richard Milne)

Hedgerows and paths

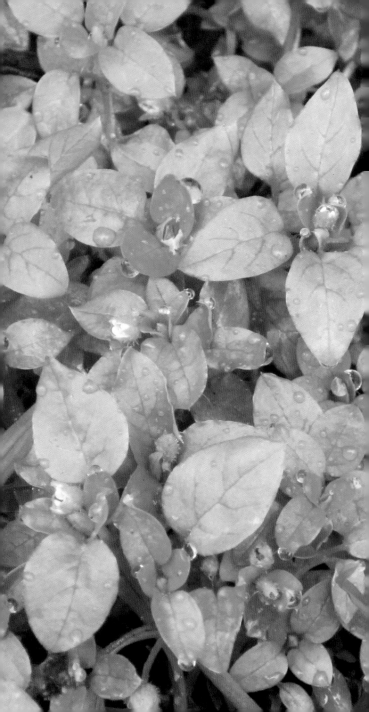

৬ Chickweed

A Staffin man told me that 'Fliodh' (Chickweed, *Stellaria media*)[40] grows in fine ground, such as a potato patch. You must use it fresh, he said: when fresh, it produces lots of sap, which is used for sciatica or rheumatism. They would chop it up and make a poultice for the knee, so that the juice penetrated the skin. As a child in the early 1960s at Da Haa of Aywick, Yell, Shetland, Hazel Gray would gather chickweed and give it to the hens 'to make their eggs good'.

Almost the commonest weed in Britain, chickweed flowers right through the year, and apart from on mountains can be found on rich soils by waysides, upper salt marshes and cultivated ground throughout Scotland, including the Northern Isles.[41]

৬ Dandelion

Dandelion (*Taraxacum officinale*), known in Gaelic as 'Beàrnan Brìde' or 'St Bride's Notched One'[42] – the leaves are notched – features in a story from the late 1930s told to me by a man from Staffin, who was told it by his mother:

> The Travelling folk used to come round the area in those days. There was a teenage boy in the village who was not well-looking; his family were concerned about him. A Travelling woman

Opposite. Chickweed

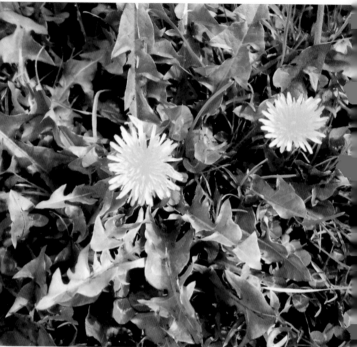

Dandelion

looked in on the family, having heard that their
boy was unwell. She asked if she could see the
boy. She looked into the boy's eyes, and after a
few moments said that she knew what was
wrong with him: he was anaemic. 'And the cure
is outside your door.' She told his mother to dig
up the dandelions by the roots, wash them, boil
them and strain the juice, which he was then to
drink. 'That shall sort out your boy!' She
promised to look in on them again in a fortnight
– and when she did, he was a changed boy.

A woman from near Talmine, Sutherland, remembers her parents in the 1950s putting the fresh milky juice of the stem of the dandelion on warts – and she still uses it today. Dandelion flowers all year round, but especially in the springtime, and flourishes in managed grassland, marshes, waysides and paths throughout Britain, including the Hebrides and the Northern Isles.[43]

☙ Docken

Docken or Dockan[44] is known as 'Cópac', 'Copag' in Gaelic. Morag Henriksen, originally from Wester Ross, relates, 'My father used to say, God was good; wherever nettles grew, dockens were never far away.'

On Lewis, copag leaves were used for nettle (p.42) stings. Agnus Maclennan, from Achmore, Lewis, said that when she was a child on the Isle of Great Bernera, she loved to eat the copag leaf. And when she went up the hill to milk the cows, she brought them fresh picked leaves of copag, which she spread out on the ground for them so that they could eat and be happy while she was milking them. A Staffin man remembered that when he was a boy in short trousers and had been stung by nettles he would rub the sting with a leaf of cópac; he might also dig it up and use the white part at the end of the root to rub on the nettle sting. On mainland Orkney, and the Isles of Stronsay and Sanday, children in the 1930s to '50s eased nettle stings and rashes by pulling off the sheath above the new leaf at the centre of the dockan and carefully catching the thick clear 'slime' that emerged from the sheath – it 'works wonders', as a number of

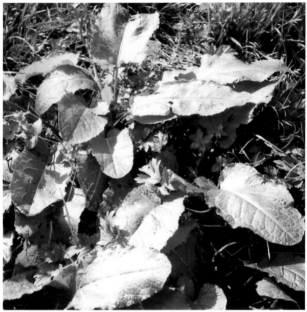

Above. Docken
Opposite. Sooracks (Heather McHaffie)

people told me in Dounby, West Mainland. Docken slime from the root was used for nettle stings in the 1930s in Lerwick, Shetland. The fresh leaf was used for stings on Yell. And in the late 1920s, on the Isle of Whalsay, the slime from the sheaf of the new leaf was put on nettle stings. Another woman in Dounby said that as a child, when playing house in Orkney, she used to gather dockan seeds for pretend 'sugar', as the reddish seeds look like big granules.

A woman from Balmaqueen, Skye, would use cópac for cuts and burns on the hands. The white part at the root's end was used as a poultice. She said it was 'a bad weed for the fields', as it grows everywhere. A man from

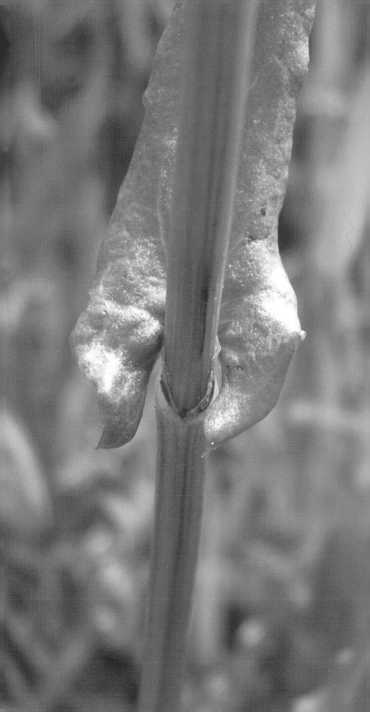

the Isle of Raasay told me that docken juice was used for thinning the blood, as well as treating boils and carbuncles. A woman from Achnahuaigh, Talmine, Sutherland, said that for a bad chest, or bad lungs, 'a poultice of the dry leaves of dockan was bandaged on the chest and left on overnight'. The fresh leaves, she remembers, were used as a poultice for bed sores, as well as for sore joints. She has also used a poultice of dockan around the abdomen for kidney cancer.

The closely related Common Sorrel, Gaelic 'Sealbhag', meaning 'Little Bitter One', is known to Scots children as 'Sooracks' because of its pleasingly sour taste.[45] (See also Crottal, p.52)

A woman in Holm, Orkney, remembers that her mother was 'always on about "sookan-sooricks"'. Sooricks were also very popular to chew on in the Shetlands, according to contributors I spoke with on Yell and mainland Shetland.

Broad Dock (*Rumex obtusifolius*, Gaelic 'Copag Leathann'[46]), which flowers from May to October, is the most common docken of roadsides throughout Scotland, preferring open areas such as field margins, ditches and waste ground. Conversely, Curled Dock is abundant in pastures. Both are found all over Britain.[47]

🙢 Hips and Haws

A friend of mine, who was evacuated during the Second World War to a boarding school at Fort Augustus, said

Opposite. Hips

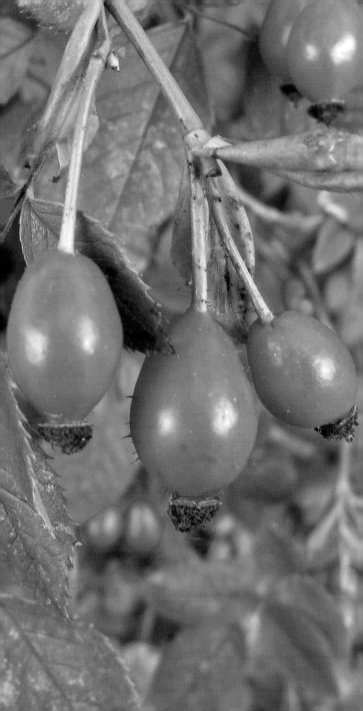

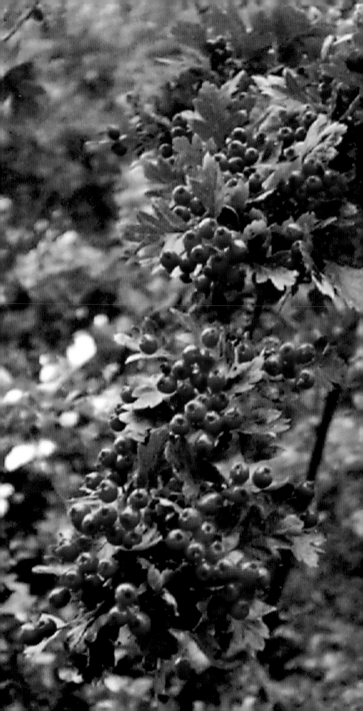

that the monks would send the boys off into the hills for walks to collect 'hips and haws' – that is, rose hips (*Rosa canina*, p.39) and haws (left) from the hawthorn (*Crataegus monogyna*) – to be made into rose hip syrup, full of vitamin C, as part of the war effort.

Morag Henriksen in Portree remembers that as a Brownie in the late 1940s in Lochcarron, Wester Ross, she was sent out to collect wild rose hips. The collected hips were then commercially boiled up into rose hip syrup. She remembers her baby sister being given this syrup.

The most common wild rose in the British Isles, *except* in Scotland, is *Rosa canina*, flowering May to July, and inhabiting hedges, scrub and woods from southern Scotland southwards. Conversely, the most common wild rose in central and northern Scotland is *R. caesia*, the Northern Dog Rose, which has larger hips than *R. canina*. Although mostly absent from the Hebrides, *R. caesia* is found on Orkney and Shetland.[48]

The common native species of hawthorn in Scotland is *Crataegus monogyna*, which flowers from late April to June, and is found widely in hedges, woodland margins and scrub up to 550 metres (including the Hebrides and the Northern Isles), but only rarely on acid sands and wet peat. *C. laevigata*, fond of clay and loam, is local in England and Wales, and flowers a week earlier than *C. monogyna*, but is absent from Scotland and Ireland.[49]

Opposite. Haws

𝒱ᴼᴬ *Nettles*

A woman from Achnahuaigh, Talmine, Sutherland, remembered her parents and grandparents using the young fresh leaves of nettles (*Urtica dioica*, Gaelic 'Deanntag', 'Feanntag'[50]) as tea – a very effective diuretic, she said. Fresh leaves were also placed in the fridge to absorb odours. The 'fat leaves' of nettles were cooked up for soup. Her husband remembered his family cooking up nettles for soup in the 1930s, and he still takes nettle soup to this day as a tonic. Another man from Culrain, Sutherland, remembers his parents gathering nettle leaves for soup in 1929.

Morag Henriksen in Portree told me of a cure she

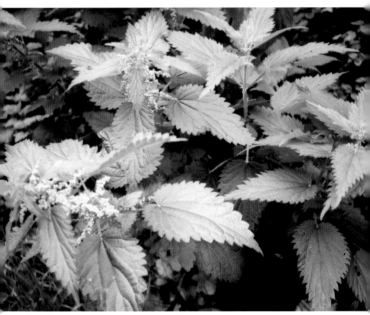

Nettles

had had from an old woman there, who had heard of it from Duncan Corbett of Uig, who had been the chauffeur to the local physician, Dr Lamont:

> There was an old man badly crippled with arthritis. A tinker at Snizort told him to take a bunch of nettles, hit the affected area several times, then bathe in the sea and leave to dry, and to repeat this twice more. Apparently the doctor came along in the car, saw the old man, told his chauffeur to stop, and pointed out to the old man that it was *his* medication that had cured him. 'Not at all,' the old man replied, 'it was the tink that cured me!'

Nettles flower from June to August, and form dense patches in shady grassy places, hedgebanks, woods and disturbed ground, especially in nitrogen-rich soil around farm buildings and villages. Generally distributed across the British Isles, they can be locally dominant.[51]

❦ *Ribwort*

Ribwort Plantain (*Plantago lanceolata*), or 'Lus na Slàn' in Skye Gaelic (also called 'Slàn-lus', 'Healing Plant'[52]), was used, according to a woman from Balmaqueen, Skye, as a remedy for whooping cough. The cones at the tip of the plant also produced a purple dye, she said. In Dumbarton in the 1950s, children made a toy gun by looping the stem of the ribwort over itself near to the seed head; they then sang a rhyme: 'Johnny had a gun and the gun was loaded, Johnny had a gun and the gun *exploded*' – and on that word they would fire the stem loop against the seed head, towards another child's toy gun. In Shetland, ribwort is called 'John's mass flooer':

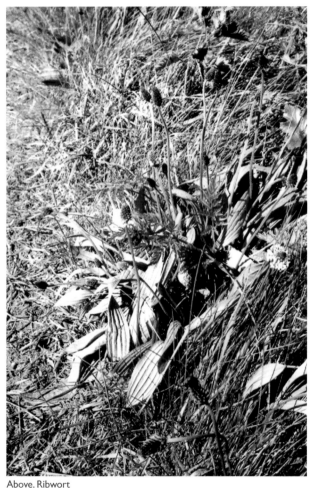

Above. Ribwort
Opposite. Rat-tail Plantain

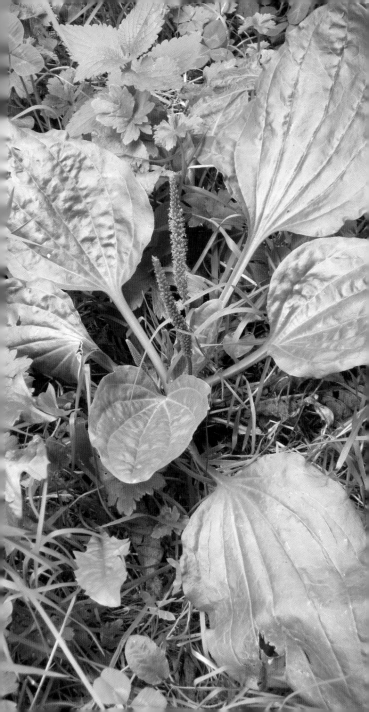

girls would pull off the stamens from the head of the
stem, put the plant under the pillow, say the name of
their true love and go to sleep. In the morning, if more
stamens had opened or appeared during the night, their
wish would come true.[53] A man from Staffin, Skye,
remembered playing a game as a boy with Lus na Slàn
where you used the stalks as swords and tried to knock
off the 'head' of your opponent's sword. If you did, you
won. A woman who grew up in Angus said that children
playing in the countryside near Arbroath in the late
1940s knew this game as 'Carl Doddies'. The man from
Staffin also remembered playing with what he called
'Cuach-Phàdraig' (that is, 'Patrick's Cup', *Plantago major*,
Rat-tail plantain, see p.45): each child grabbed hold of
one end of the leaf and pulled, and the one with more
'strings' left in his hand was the winner.

Ribwort, flowering in spring and early summer, is
common throughout Britain, where it flourishes in
grassy places. Rat-tail plantain, flowering in summer, is
very widespread in well-trodden places in Scotland (and
the rest of Britain) by roadsides, waste ground, lawns,
fields and gardens.[54]

✿ Thistle

A woman remembers that when she was a child in the
1960s in Holm, West Mainland, Orkney, her father
would 'get thistle cheese' by peeling the head of a
purple-flowering scotch thistle to reveal a white 'peedie

Opposite. Melancholy thistle (Heather McHaffie)

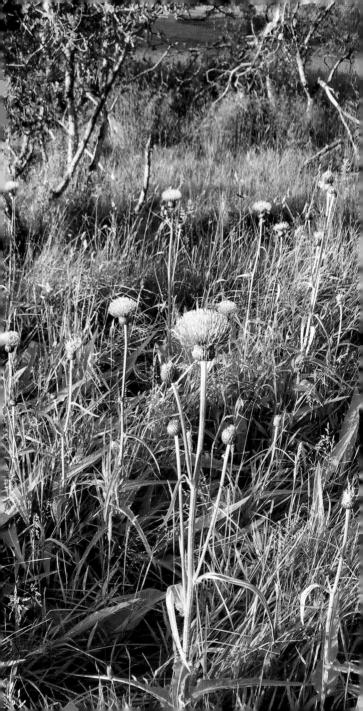

cheese' inside. Her father would take a bite of it, and
then give her a bite of it, in turns. By her description of
the plant, I take this to be the Melancholy Thistle
(*Cirsium helenioides*)[55] that flowers in July and August
by streams, in damp grassland, open woods and scrub,
and in the hills; it is found in the Orkneys, as well as
the north and west Highlands and the Hebrides, but is
mostly absent south of the border.[56]

Hillsides and moorland

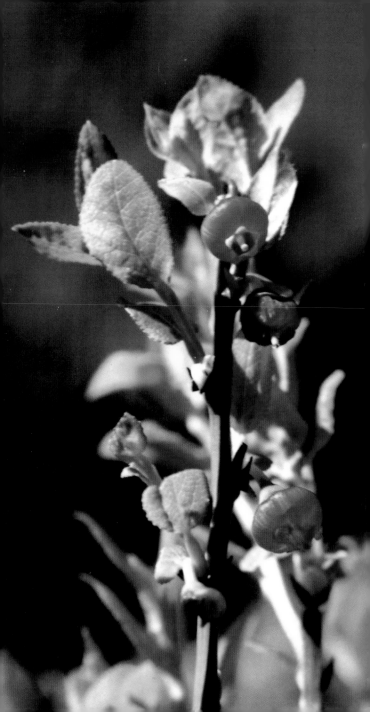

ஃ Blaeberries

A woman in Staffin said that blaeberries (*Vaccinium myrtillus*, Gaelic 'Coara-mhitheag'[57]) would turn your tongue dark blue when you ate them. A woman from Uig on Skye remembered that after the Second World War she gathered blaeberries, near Dunkeld in Perthshire, to make a tart, but that they wouldn't keep for jam.

In Talmine, Sutherland, blaeberries were collected from the hillside and made into jam; there was always a jar in the cupboard against colds, said a woman from Achnahuaigh, Melness. She remembers her parents and grandparents making it before the Second World War. Mary Beith told me that she was told by the late Hugh MacDonald of Melness, who had it from his parents and grandparents, that the berries, known locally in Sutherland as 'Fiagag' or 'Fiadhag', were prepared as a

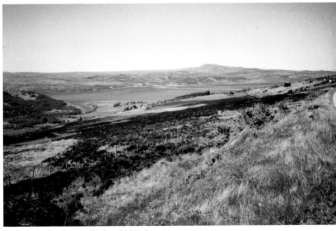

Opposite. Blaeberry (Richard Milne)
Above. Kyle of Tongue, Sutherland

tonic, and used for kidney and bladder stones, for stomach troubles, and for the eyes. Agnus Maclennan told me that on the Isle of Great Bernera, Lewis, in the 1930s, children ate blaeberries, called 'Curach Mheig',[58] straight off the bushes as a delicacy; they grew near the heather, quite close to the shoreline.

Blaeberry flowers from April to June, and occurs on acid soil in open woods and moors up to 1,220 metres; on mountains above the heather line it is dominant, perhaps because it tolerates shade and exposure better than heather (p.57). It is common throughout Scotland, but mostly absent from south-east and central England.[59]

৶৹ *Brambles*

Brambles (*Rubus fruticosus*), known in Skye Gaelic as 'Smior dues',[60] were gathered to make jam, according to a woman from Balmaqueen. Brambles are found throughout Scotland, but are scattered in the Highlands and Islands, rare in Orkney, and absent from Shetland. Flowering from May to November, they grow in woods, roadsides and bushy places.[61]

৶৹ *Crottal*

Crottal or crottle (Gaelic 'crotal', *Parmelia* spp.[62]) is a dye-producing lichen. Around the Isle of Great Bernera,

Opposite. Brambles

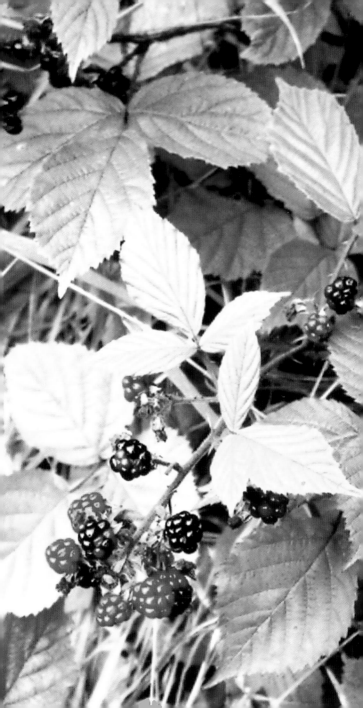

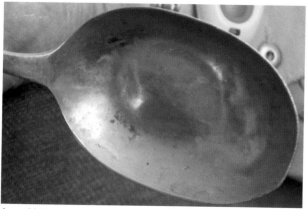

Agnus Maclennan's crottal spoon

Lewis, crottal refers specifically to a greyish-brown lichen which produces a rich brown colour when making the tweed.

Agnus Maclennan, who was brought up in Kirkibost, Great Bernera, in the 1930s, showed me a 'crottal spoon' (above); as a child she only ever used it for scraping the crottal off the rocks on the island. They gave the crottal they had collected to the crofter next door, who made the tweed. As children, they also used to have to 'pee in a pot', as urine was used for 'waulking the tweed'.

Mòr Macleod, who was born at the beginning of the First World War on a croft in a hamlet near Earshader on Lewis, just opposite Great Bernera, told me that as the sheep were shorn in June and July, the crottal had to be ready for the dyeing of the fleeces by August. The crottal was scraped off the rocks out on the moor. It dyes the wool fleeces 'a nice colour of brown'. There were four crofts in the hamlet, with a burn running down between them. A large boiler was set up next to the burn, and a peat fire would be laid under it. Inside the boiler they first put a layer of crottal, then a layer of fleece, then crottal, and so on until the boiler was nearly full. On the top of these layers they put the leaves of the 'sealbhag', the sorrel (*Rumex acetosa,* see Docken, p.35), as these were used to fix the dye. Then water from the burn was added until the boiler was full. A wooden lid was fitted to the top, and a large stone was placed on the lid to hold it down. They kept the peat fire going under the boiler all day, and then in the evening they removed the lid and let the fire die down overnight. In the morning, every-

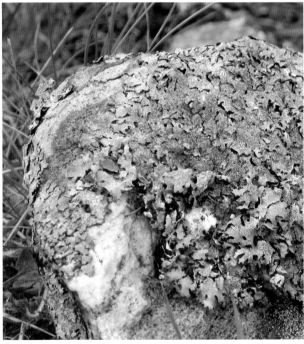

Crottal

thing had cooled off. They pulled the fleeces out of the boiler, shook the crottal off them, and washed them in a pool in the burn. Then they would hang the fleeces to dry on the wall. From the crofts, the finished fleeces were sent to the mill in Stornoway, where they were spun into yarn. The yarn was then sent back to Earshader, where there were quite a few weavers of tweed; the weavers worked on big wooden looms with four pedals. This was in the 1920s.

🍃 Crowberry

Hazel Gray told me that in Aywick, Yell, Shetland, as soon as the end of July came in, it was berry time, and all the kids would go up into the hills to gather the 'berry hedder' (the local name for the crowberry, *Empetrum nigrum*; in Shetland dialect hedder = heather) to eat them straight off the bush. They turned your tongue purple, and were slightly bitter: 'if you ate too many, you got a sore belly'. As a child in the 1920s and '30s, Charlie Johnson of Quarff, Shetland, went up on the hills in late July to eat the berries off the bush. His friend Nicol Stove remembers eating them raw in the 1930s and '40s in Sandwick, Shetland, and collecting them in a pail to be made into jam by his mother. For jam, he said, you boil the berries with sugar; but the jam didn't last long, as they put it on bannocks and ate it all up.

The crowberry flowers in May and June, and is found on moors, as well as the more dry areas of blanket bogs. While common in Scotland, the north of England and Wales, it is rare or absent in the south of England.[63]

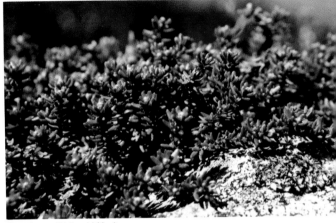

Crowberry (Richard Milne)

❧ *Heather*

A man in Talmine, Sutherland, said that between the wars he remembers watching a heather bed being made. The heather bed, he added, is mentioned in a Gaelic song by the 18th-century Sutherland bard Rob Donn. The heather (*Calluna vulgaris*, Gaelic 'Fraoch'[64]) needed to come from 'hard hills' or by the side of a burn. It was cut evenly – from eight to twelve inches high – made to stand upright, packed in tightly, tied, and then covered with a dried hide. It would last for many years. It made an excellent mattress, he said, and was much favoured by the old folks for a good sleep. Over it you placed a chaff (p.6) mattress. Another man, from Altandubh, Wester Ross, told me that he remembers his father, a carpenter (born in 1860), describing to his sons how a heather bed was constructed. The plants were cut just above the roots, placed flower-side up in a box frame,

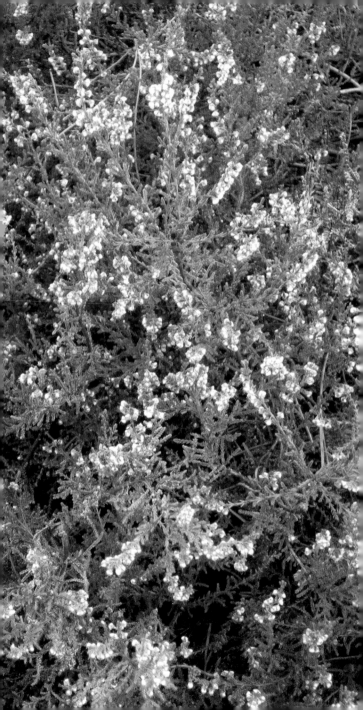

and then packed in as tightly as possible until the frame was filled. It was very pleasant to sleep on, he said.

Heather is found on acid soils throughout the British Isles, especially heaths, bogs, moors, fixed dunes and open woods. A favourite food of the red grouse, it flowers from July to September, and may be dominant on moorlands in a narrow zone above the mountain treeline.[65]

Primrose

Mòr Macleod, of Brue, Lewis, told me that primrose leaves (*Primula vulgaris,* Gaelic 'Sòbrach'[66]) were used for infected cuts in Earshader, Lewis, in the 1920s. The leaves, available in spring and summer, were only ever used fresh as a poultice, she said. 'You found them quite often in bunches by the burn, on moist ground.'

In Kirkibost on the Isle of Great Bernera, Lewis, in the early summer of 1943, when Agnus Maclennan was ten, she told me that she got boils on her leg: 'they were itchy and wouldn't heal up'. The district nurse on Great Bernera advised Agnus' mother that she should take the child to the doctor. The doctor was based at Uig on Lewis, but once a week he came to the community hall at Breclate (Breacleite) on Great Bernera. When he saw the boils, he told them that Agnus had 'droch fhuil'.[67] He prescribed a three-part treatment over three months, which included eating raw lamb's liver each day, taking a penny-piece's weight of powdered sulphur in a

Opposite. Heather

teaspoon three times a day, and putting a poultice of fresh primrose leaves on the leg, with the dressing to be changed each day. The primrose leaves had to be gathered fresh daily from two crofts away, where there was a hillock with a burn running beside it: 'you could see their yellow flowers close to the ground'. The 'veiny' underside of the leaf was placed over the top of the boils on Agnus' leg, and then over this a bandage made of pillowcase material was wrapped around it. After a few weeks of this treatment, the leg started to heal. 'It was obvious,' said Agnus. 'The wound came together. The veiny side of the leaf had drawn the pus away.' Now that there was no longer any infection, the softer, top side of the primrose leaf was used, face down, over the wound, to help complete the healing. Her mother continued to change the poultice daily until the leg was completely healed. It took three months from start to finish, and the cure became well known across the Isle of Lewis.

Primrose, which flowers from March to May (and even earlier in milder locales), is found throughout Scotland, including the Hebrides and the Northern Isles, in hedgebanks, woods, open grassy places and sea cliffs; while formerly common in Britain, it is now scarce or virtually extinct near large towns because of over-picking.[68]

❧ Roseroot

'Lus nan Laoch', 'The Warrior's Plant', is probably *Sedum rosea*.[69] While its Gaelic name sounds similar to that of Bog Bean ('Lus-na-Laogh' or 'Lus-na-Laoich'), 'The

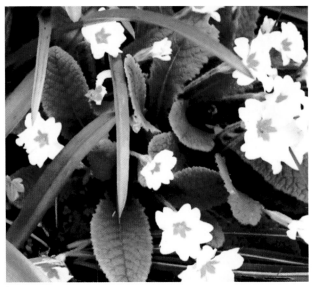

Primrose

Warrior's Plant' is nothing like it, as it is found in a completely different habitat to that of Bog Bean (p.65), or for that matter Golden Saxifrage ('Lus nan Laogh', see below). A woman in Staffin on Skye said that Flora MacInnes had told her in 1998 that the reason it was called 'The Warrior's Plant' was because you had to climb up a cliff to get at it. This plant, which she said was used for ulcers, had evergreen leaves, with 'a wee tiny creamy berry'. She thought it was also called 'The Calves' Plant', because it gave you strong calves to get up to it. But according to Scott, the 'Plant of the Calves', 'Lus nan Laogh', is a form of Golden Saxifrage (*Chrysosplenium oppositifolium*), which grows on wet ground, near springs and streams, throughout Scotland; a perennial (not an evergreen), it forms a loose mat of stems with pale green

opposite pairs of leaves, petal-less flowers but with four
or five yellow sepals frilled by bright green bracts.[70]

Now Scott[71] identifies the Gaelic 'Lus nan Laoch'
('The Heroes' Plant') as Roseroot, which grows on coastal
cliffs and in mountains. An evergreen with bluish, flat
leaves, it has a fleshy rootstock that smells of rose when
cut. The flower heads are rounded, greenish-yellow and
have four-petalled flowers from May to August; it is
common in crevices of sea cliffs in western Scotland and
Ireland.[72] Roseroot was thought to be popular with the
Vikings, who found that it gave them greater 'mental and
physical endurance'.[73] Of old, Vikings were frequent
visitors to the Hebrides, and one might speculate an
association with 'Warriors'. The closely related Houseleek
(*Sempervivum tectorum*) has a long tradition of use,
especially for burns and scalds. A woman on Iona told
me she remembered that in the late 1940s in East
Yorkshire her aunt treated her for a bee sting with the cut
side of a houseleek that grew in her garden rockery. In
Sweden, it was used to preserve the roofs of houses.[74]

Roseroot (Richard Milne)

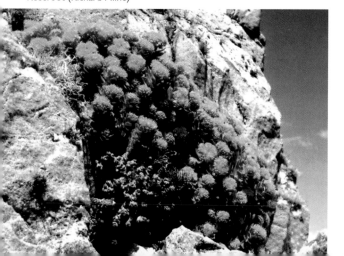

Lochs, bogs and wells

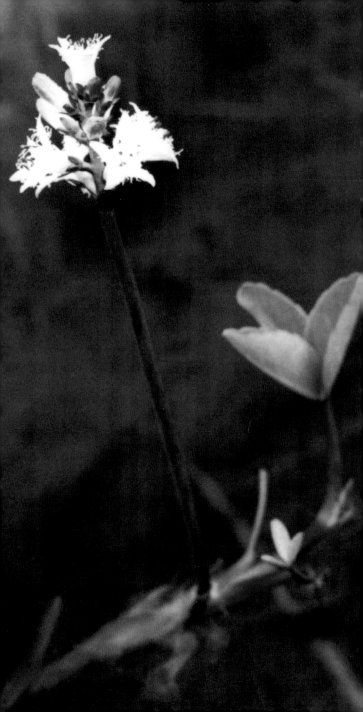

ঙৡ *Bog Bean*

Bog Bean (*Menyanthes trifoliata*) is a beautiful loch-side plant known in Skye Gaelic as 'Trì-bhileach' ('Three-leaved One'); on Lewis and elsewhere in the Highlands and Islands, it is called 'Lus-na-Laogh' or 'Lus-na-Laoich'.[75] Mary Beith told me of a man in Lewis who made his own bog bean tonic and drank it regularly.

According to Mary, it tastes 'utterly foul'; she related to me the following story about him:

> Two elderly sisters came to him on behalf of a third sister who was suffering from a skin rash. Orthodox medicine had been unable to help her. They asked him for some bog bean tonic so

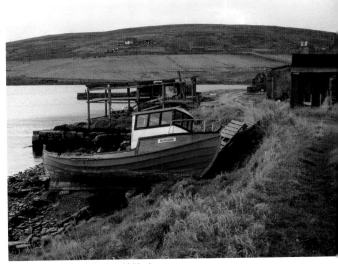

Opposite. Bog Bean (Richard Milne)
Above. Seafield, Mid Yell, Shetland

that they could take it to her. They wanted to pay
him, but he refused to take any money. He sent
them off with the tonic. Two weeks later they
came back, full of smiles, and carrying a box of
chocolates and two packets of cigarettes for him.
Their sister had been completely cured of her
complaint.

A man in Staffin, Skye, said that trì-bhileach grows in
abundance in the lochs about Staffin. He told me this
story from the 1940s:

An old man in Stenschol, Staffin, was suffering
from duodenal ulcers. A woman in nearby
Flodigarry gathered leaves growing in the loch;
she washed, sliced and boiled them, strained the
juice, and bottled it. She told him to take one
eggcup-ful of the juice each day. He did this and
was no longer troubled by the ulcers.

A woman in Uig, Skye, passed on to me a recipe for bog
bean tonic (lus-na-laogh) that came from Lochs, on the
Isle of Lewis. Here the tonic is recommended for
carbuncles: 'Take twenty stems of the flowers, found at
the edge of freshwater lochs; clean for twelve hours in
six pints water. Dispose of stems; sieve water twice
through a clean cloth. Bottle. Ready to drink. Take a
small glass each day until the carbuncle disappears.'
    This last remedy is from a woman in Portree, Skye:
the leaves of the plant were gathered before they flower,
and then dried. Once the leaves were dry, you crumpled
the leaves and kept them in a tight tin to use as tea. They

were said to be very bitter but excellent, and were used by the woman's grandfather and family regularly.

Flowering in May and June, bog bean is found throughout Britain in ponds, wet bogs and at the edges of shallow lochs, especially in the west of Scotland, the Hebrides, and the Northern Isles.[76]

Bog Cotton

A man from Cunningsburgh, Shetland, remembered that during the Second World War, bog cotton (*Eriophorum angustifolium*) was collected on mainland Shetland for use as a wound dressing. Common Cotton-grass, as it is also known, flowers in May and June in wet acid places.[77]

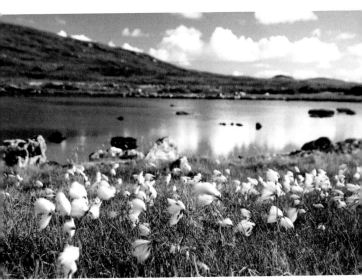

Bog Cotton (Richard Milne)

℘ *Bog Myrtle*

A man from Raasay told me that Bog Myrtle (*Myrica gale*, Gaelic 'Roid'[78]) was hung up in the house; it had a pleasant smell, he said. He also told me that a leaf of the plant was added to a pot of soup, much as we would use a bay leaf. Bog myrtle grows in wet heathland and bogs, to 550 metres, and flowers in April and May. It occurs locally throughout Britain, but in Scotland it is more frequent in the south-west, the Highlands and Islands, and Orkney.[79]

Bog Myrtle

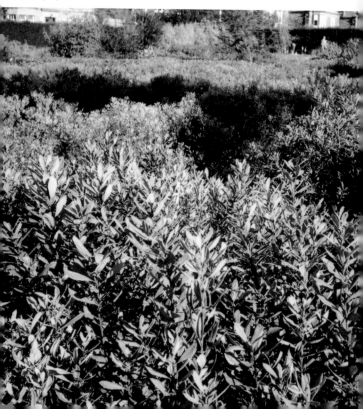

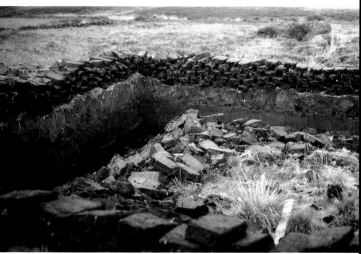

Peat, North Uist (Heather McHaffie)

❧ Peat

A woman from Achnahuaigh, Sutherland, recalled that when her grandparents and parents were young, before the World Wars, they would prepare themselves before going out to a dance at night by taking peat and mud and 'clarting' it on their faces. The pack was left on for ten minutes, and then washed off. Their skin would look brightened and beautiful.

Peat is formed in bogs from mosses; *Sphagnum palustre* is a key species in peat formation. However, there are thirty-five recognised species of sphagnum moss (p.71) in Britain, all of which could be converted to peat: the species present depend on the pH of the water in the blanket bog, and how dry the moorland is.[80]

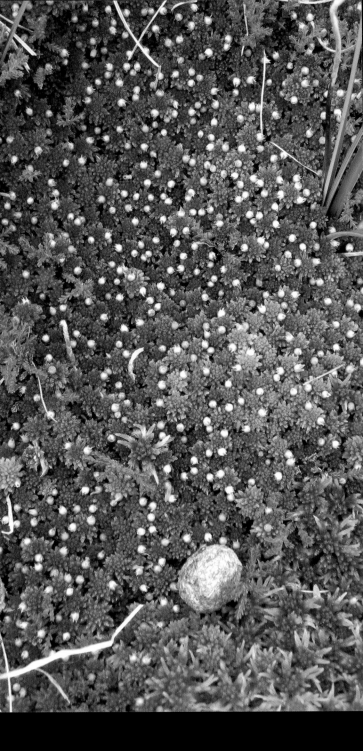

𝒫ᴥ *Sphagnum moss*

During the war (1939–41), a friend of mine was evacuated to the school at Fort Augustus. The boys at the school were sent up into the hills to collect sphagnum moss (Gaelic 'còinneach dhearg'[81]). The dried moss would then be packed into tins at Red Cross centres, where it would in turn be sent off to the Front for use in field-dressing kits. A woman from St Andrews remembers packing sphagnum moss into tins for the Red Cross at the Younger Hall during the Second World War. An Edinburgh woman said that in the early 1940s she was sent out to Balerno by bus to gather 'the red moss' for the war effort. A man from Lochnell, Argyll, told me that sphagnum moss was greatly used during the First World War. A man from Altandubh said that in 1914, when he was seven, he was sent by his mother, who was the schoolteacher, to collect both green moss and red moss. The red moss was the best, he said. The red moss was separated out, and then both sorts were spread out to dry in the classroom. The dried moss was packed into special labelled bags that were sent on to the Front. Mòr Macleod of Brue, Lewis, told me that during the Second World War, when she was the district nurse for the villages in and around Brue, cotton wool was hard to get – indeed, everything was hard to get. She remembered that the red sphagnum moss was collected in bags all round that area and, through the Red Cross, it was sent out to the hospitals.

Several women in Dounby, Orkney, vividly remem-

Opposite. Sphagnum moss (Heather McHaffie)

bered that in 1939–40 Lady Dalrymple, dressed in
tweeds, came to the schools at Dounby and Harray to
tell the children how sphagnum moss would be used for
wound dressings in the war. They said that during her
visit she stayed at Balfour Castle on the Isle of Shapinsay.
One of them remembered that her friend's mother went
up to Glims Moss, on the road to Evie, to gather up the
moss in her pony cart. Once the cart was full, she drove
it back down to the school in Dounby to be sorted out
by members of the Scottish Womens' Rural Institute.

In the last years of the First World War, 'there was a
great demand for the moss as a dressing for soldiers'
wounds', according to Helen Jamieson, who lived at the
time in Gossabrough, Yell, Shetland. 'My sisters and me
and three elder girls, we went to a hill where there was a
lot of this moss in a damp place at the back of the hill. It
was all yellow moss.' The girls filled two and a half huge
bags full of the moss, then took it to the pier where the
steamer landed at Gossabrough. A man from Quarff,
Shetland, who was born in 1919, remembers his mother
telling him that she and her neighbours had collected
the yellow moss in a bag from the hills around Quarff
during the First World War to be used for the soldiers'
wounds.

Morag Henriksen of Portree, Skye, told me that
sphagnum moss is 'the best thing for cleaning your
hands after peat cutting. It feels lovely on your skin'; her
father had told her this when she was a child in
Lochcarron, Wester Ross.

Sphagnum moss absorbs sixty times its weight in
water.[82] It grows in peat bogs and lime-free wet spots,
moors and mountains, often forming clumps; and it is

found throughout Scotland, as well as in Ireland, Wales, Yorkshire, the Lake District, Devon and the Wye Valley.[83]

❧ *Watercress*

A Staffin man remembered that he would go up to a 'well' (a spring) surrounded by limestone where he would gather 'Biolaire' (*Nasturtium officinale*, watercress).[84] 'Many a time I would chew it as a boy,' he said. 'It had a pleasant taste.' Gaelic 'Biolair' refers to many cresses, according to Dwelly; while Scott suggests that it may refer to an old word for water.[85] The fact that it was

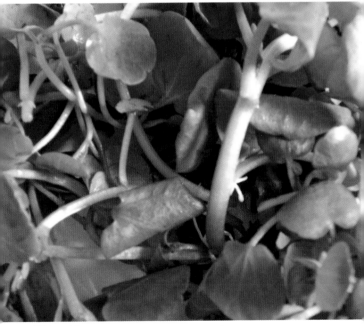

Watercress

a limestone well is significant; the sheep liver fluke, which usually infests watercress, hates limestone.[86]

A man in Achnahuaigh, Sutherland, collects watercress in the springtime from the burn near his house, as his family has done since the 1930s. He uses watercress to remove toxins from the body. To prepare it, he washes it first with mild bleach or iodine (to remove the flukes), and then washes it well again to remove the bleach. He takes it regularly.

Flowering from May to October, watercress grows in shallow, flowing fresh water near limestone. It is commonly found in lowland Britain, including the Hebrides, Orkney and Shetland, but is absent from parts of the north and west Highlands.[87]

Seashore

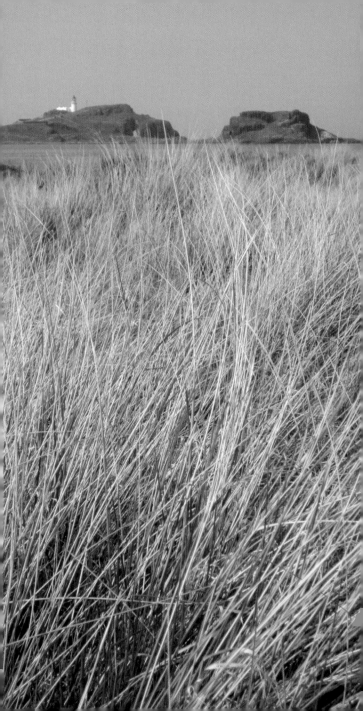

❧ *Broad Bent*

Jimmy Work, of Scousburgh, Dunrossness, Shetland, makes woven baskets from 'broad bent', also called 'seablue grass' or marram grass (*Ammophila arenaria*), that he collects from the dunes down on Scousburgh Beach. The pattern of the weave is similar to that which he uses for making his oat straw baskets (Oat Straw, p.14).

A stout, tall plant, marram helps bind the dunes with its rootstock. Flowering in July and August, it is widespread along British coasts.[88]

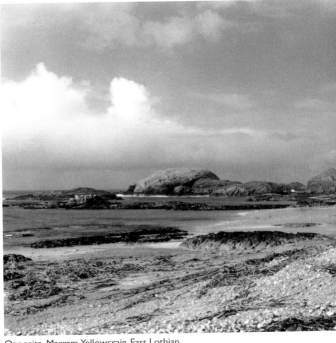

Opposite. Marram, Yellowcraig, East Lothian
Above. Iona, Port of the White Stones

❧ *Carrageen*

A woman in Staffin, Skye, said that 'Careagan' (*Chondrus crispus*, carrageen)[89] is best gathered in August. 'It grows on the rocks of the lower foreshore. You must wait for a very low ebb tide to collect it. It is very dark when wet.' Her friend added that careagan is known as the 'mother of the dulse' because the dulse grows on top of it on the rocks. After gathering the careagan, it is bleached by placing it on sheets of newspaper, weighted down with stones, on top of the shed roof, to dry out in the sun. To make careagan pudding, she told me, take a good pinch of dried careagan and put it into a little water; boil it ten minutes. Then add milk and boil another ten minutes.

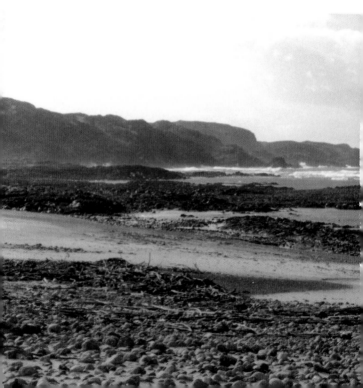

Sieve the mixture, and serve with cream or a little jelly. 'Beautiful,' she said, 'like a cornflour pudding. It is easy on the stomach, so very good for anybody with stomach trouble. Add just a little sugar to it.'

Mòr Macleod said that in Earshader, Lewis, they went out in a very low tide in August and September, and gathered the 'cairgein' off the rocks. On a nice day they washed it and spread it out to dry on top of clean linen. Once it was dry, they could store it for using through the year. Both in Earshader and on the Isle of Great Bernera, Lewis, the method of cooking it was to put it in the pot with cold milk, then bring it just to the

Iona, Port of Andrew's Headland

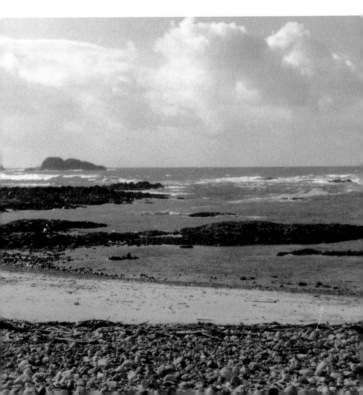

point where the milk was beginning to scald, stirring it all the time. Then it was sieved into a plate; as it cooled, it became 'like jelly or junket'. 'You give it to those who had sore stomachs, indigestion of any kind, or ulcers, especially duodenal ulcers. It was very soothing.' Carrageen is commonly found at low tide on North Atlantic seashores.[90]

🙞 Dulse

Like Carrageen (p.78), Dulse (*Palmaria palmata;* Gaelic 'duleasg', 'duileasg'[91]) has many uses. A Staffin man told me that you can collect dulse all year long. You don't dry it first, he said, but wash it before chopping it up well. He and his friend from Raasay both like dulse soup, as well as careagan pudding. A woman in Staffin makes dulse soup, which is full of iron and other minerals: she cooks the dulse with the shank bone of a salt ham, or a mutton bone, together with onion and pearl barley. Her friend from Balmaqueen adds a little oatmeal to the soup about ten minutes before the end of cooking.

A man from Sutherland said that, as a boy in the 1920s in Talmine, after school he and his friends would go crabbing on the rocks by the shore, pick dulse, rinse it in the tide pools and eat it straight away. Later on, they might toast it on a stick over a fire and then eat it. He also collected the dulse from the beach, and afterwards it was dried and cooked into a pudding by his mother.

A woman from Achnahuaigh in Sutherland told me that dulse made into a pudding was 'a great pick-me-up' when one was ill or convalescent; her mother loved it, and asked for it when she was ill. Her husband also remembers his mother making it. The plant strips were collected and then hung up to dry inside. Her mother used it continuously from before the First World War, and my informant still makes it. A man from Altandubh, Wester Ross, also liked dulse very much, and remembers his mother making it into a pudding before the First World War when he was a wee boy.

Mòr Macleod of Brue, Lewis, said that you can get 'duileasg' all year round there, unlike the 'cairgein'. Agnus Maclennan told me that on the Isle of Great Bernera they would eat it raw – it was very chewy – or they would bring it into the house, where it was put into cold water with a pinch of salt and brought to the boil, like soup. She remembered them saying that it helped the digestion.

A man from Portree told me that in 1950, when he was a wee boy on holiday in Braes, Aird, Skye, he used to collect dulse with his father from the lower foreshore rocks and put it into the basket, under the watchful eye of their seventy year old neighbour, Angus MacDonald, who was wanting the dulse, but was no longer able to climb out on the rocks. The man remembered his father and Angus MacDonald speaking of the recipe for making dulse soup for the 'rheumatics' (containing cooked barley, broth from a mutton shank or a ham bone, and the dulse). This recipe, they said, was passed on to the folk there from the 'spey wife' who used to live on that very beach three hundred years earlier, in a house below the high-tide mark (so that she didn't have to pay rates). When he was a boy, the man said, you could still see the ruins of her cottage on the beach.

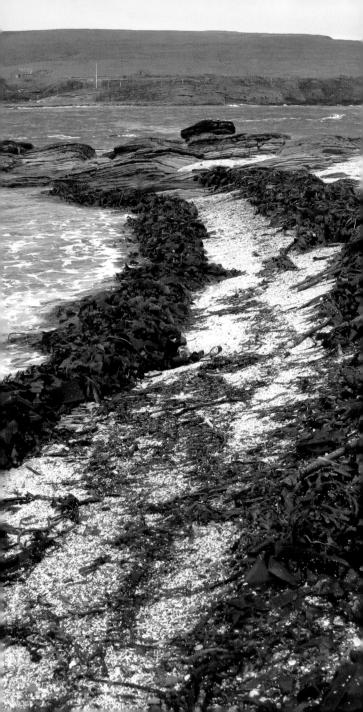

℘ *Fucus*

'Feamainn-chìrean' (Channelled Fucus,[92] *Pelvetia canaliculata*) is full of iron, according to a man from the Isle of Raasay. They would feed it to the cattle all winter, and the cattle loved it. He had heard during the Second World War from a Swedish girl that in Sweden this seaweed is mixed with oatmeal, fried up and served as a delicacy; but he had never tried it.

His friend from Staffin added that each seaweed has its own place on the shoreline: first the feamainn-chìrean, which is golden in colour, then further down the bladderwrack seaweed, then the dulse (p.80), and at the lowest ebb the careagan (Carrageen, p.78).

Helen Jamieson, who was born before the First World War, remembers using seaweed as manure on her croft at Gossabrough, East Yell, Shetland. She grew Shetland oats, potatoes, turnips and Shetland kale on the croft. She also fed seaweed to the sheep and cows. After a big storm, she remembered, there was a certain seaweed that came ashore: it had a long solid strip in the middle, that was frilly around the edge: 'Folk would gather this, dry it and store it in the kist to eat in time of famine.' According to Hazel Gray, at her childhood home of Da Haa of Aywick, Yell, 'it was always deemed sensible to allow your sheep on the beach in the winter, not only for the health of the sheep, but for the flavour of the meat'. At Sandwick, Shetland, Nicol Stove remembers collecting the 'tang'[93] from the seashore to use as manure on the croft; he also remembers that when he was a boy

Opposite. Brough of Birsay, Orkney

during the Second World War their Icelandic horse loved
to go on the beach in winter to eat the tang.

Trees and woodland

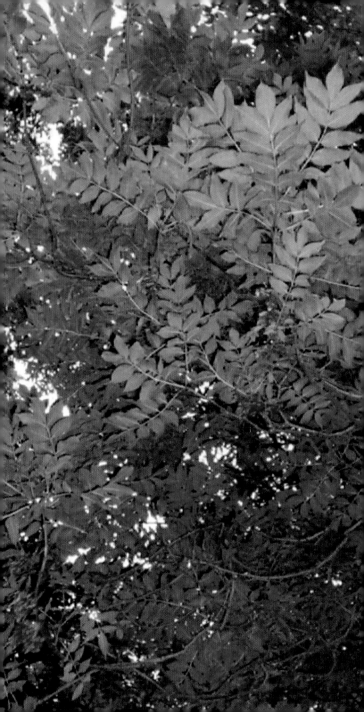

ৎঽ *Ash Tree*

A man from Staffin told me that the leaves of the Ash (*Fraxinus excelsior*[94], Gaelic 'uinnseann'[95]) were made into a poultice for the bites of adders.

A woman now living in Edinburgh shared a story about the ash from her childhood in the late 1940s in rural County Galway, Ireland. 'In those days in the country, there were many tinkers about. You always gave the tinkers something when they called at the door. And there was always a peat fire burning on the hearth. One day – I was maybe three or four – I had a terrible sore ear, and was crying because it hurt badly. A tinker woman came to the door, but my mother was distracted, and kept saying over and over, "I must see to the child." The woman asked what was wrong with me, and my

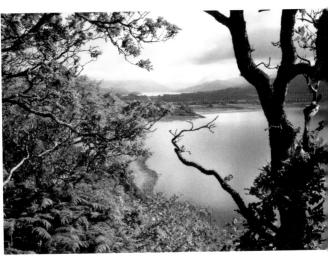

Opposite. Ash Tree
Above. Lochnell, Argyll

mother told her. She then told my mother to "take the ash plant, put it in the white part of the fire, wait for the sap to come out the other end, collect it in a spoon, and put it in the child's ear". My mother did this, and I've never had another earache.'

Mary Beith reports a story from the Highlands[96] where the instructions are almost identical to the Galway story above, but the spoonful of sap is given to a newborn child as its first taste of food.

The ash, which flowers in April and May, is commonly found in woods and hedges, on chalk soils, especially in damp parts, throughout the British Isles; less frequently it may be found on acid soil and in drier regions.[97]

🙟 Bay Willow

Bay Willow (*Salix pentandra*[98]) features in a story I was told by a woman in Melness, Sutherland. Twenty years or so ago, she was suffering from arthritis that caused great pain in her neck, leaving her feeling depleted and worn down. The cause of the pain and fatigue was yet undiagnosed: it subsequently turned out that spondylitis had led to the collapse of a vertebra, which was nipping the carotid artery. But at the time she didn't know this. She took to walking around the glen where she lived, a mile or so a day, just to keep moving. One day on her walk, she came to a tree, and stopped in front of it. She looked at the tree, and a peaceful feeling descended over

Opposite. Bay Willow

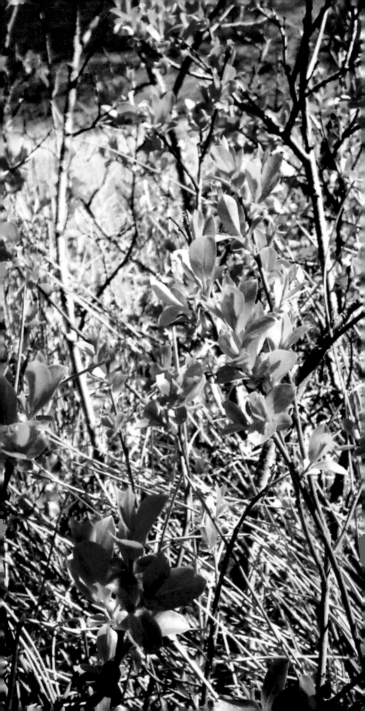

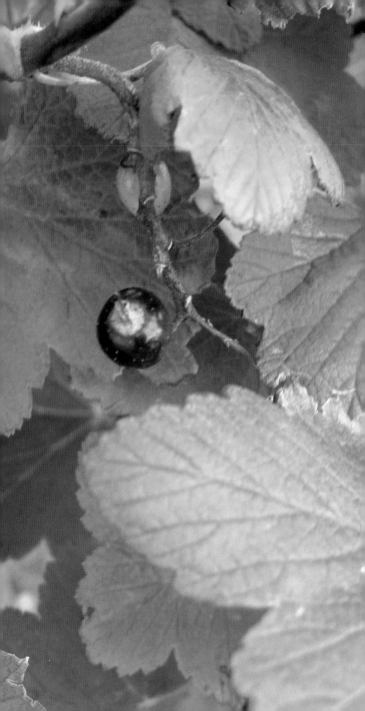

her. She found herself saying aloud, 'You're a healing tree.' It was a turning point. She took a sprig of the tree, put it in her pocket and carried it about with her. At night she put it under her pillow. Every few weeks she replaced the sprig with a fresh one. She found that it restored her, giving her hope that she would eventually be well again. Some years later, the family dog, a collie called Meg, was arthritic and declining. She wanted to bring Meg into the kitchen, but the dog wouldn't let anyone move her from the front room. In desperation, she got her grandchildren to go to the 'Healing Tree' to collect a sprig. They then tied this sprig with string around the dog's neck, so that it was under her ear. After about ten minutes, Meg got up and walked into the kitchen – and lived for another year.

Bay willow flowers in May and June, and grows on wet ground, near fresh water, in fens and wet woods, up to 460 metres; in Scotland it is mostly absent from the Highlands and Islands and the Grampians, as well as the south of England, but it may be found in the north of England, North Wales and Northern Ireland, although it is not common.[99]

❧ Black Currant

A woman from Birsay, Orkney, recalled how when she was a child, during the Second World War, her grandmother made black currant jam. If you had a sore throat, she said, you were given a spoonful of the jam, and it

Opposite. Black Currant

worked – 'maybe not every time'. Her grandmother, also from Birsay, was born around 1870.

On the Isle of Great Bernera, Lewis, black currants grew wild by the shore, in spite of the salt winds from the Atlantic, and were transplanted into croft gardens. The fruits were made into jam or eaten with cream. Agnus Maclennan, brought up in Kirkibost on Great Bernera, told me that a hot drink, 'good for opening tubes and clearing the chest', was made as follows: 'Boil black currants until mushy, mash them with a spoon, put some in a glass, pour boiling water on it, let it cool a bit, then while still quite hot, gargle with it and then swallow it.'

Black currant (*Ribes nigrum*), which flowers in April and May, is found growing wild especially by streams, in damp woods and hedges throughout Britain, including Orkney; it may be bird-sown in drier places.[100]

🍃 Gooseberry

Gooseberry bushes (*Ribes uva-crispa*) grew wild near the shore on the Isle of Great Bernera, Lewis, and were transplanted, like the black currants above, into croft gardens. Agnus Maclennan remembered that as a child in the 1930s in Kirkibost, Great Bernera, they used to eat the gooseberries – said to be 'good for constipation' – with cream from their own cow. Gooseberry flowers from March to May, and is widely found in woods, hedges and scrub (often bird-sown), but may be native in damp woods; it is found on Skye, but is scarce or absent elsewhere in the Hebrides.[101]

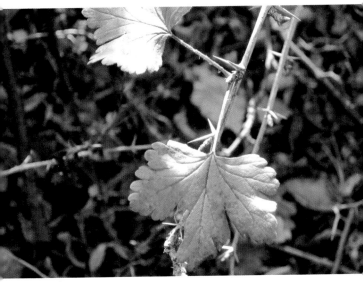

Gooseberry

Honeysuckle

Honeysuckle (*Lonicera periclymenum*), known in Gaelic as 'Feìthlean', 'Iochd slàinte', 'Iadh-shlat' ('Twig that Surrounds') or 'Lus na Meala' ('Honey Plant'),[102] was mentioned by three contributors in Staffin, on the Isle of Skye, as a remedy for asthma: you chopped it down, boiled it in water, and then took the water as for tea. Mary Beith, of Melness, Sutherland, told me how, after a neighbour's cat came to stay, she experienced severe asthma. None of her conventional inhalers worked. As it was a Saturday evening, she was unable to get to the doctor, and was too remote for a hospital. In desperation, she tried a remedy she had heard about that was traditional in Sutherland. She went to her garden and

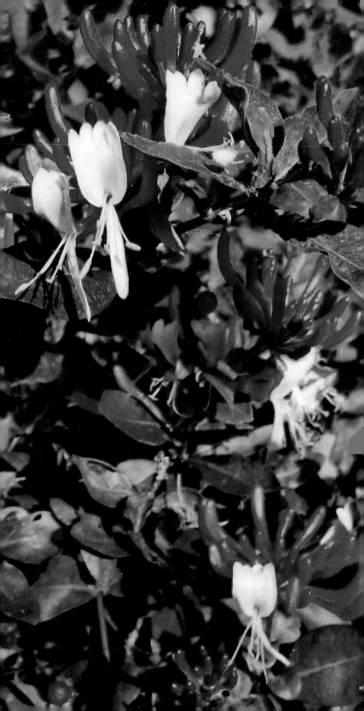

picked the honeysuckle flowers (even in September there were still some left). These she then steeped in hot water, and drank the infusion. Her throat and chest cleared completely in less than twenty minutes. Her neighbour brought a big bag full of the flowers, with which she made a strong infusion, and then froze as ice cubes for future use. She now swears by it.

Honeysuckle flowers from June to September, and grows on tree trunks, shady rocks, scrub and hedgerows up to 600 metres. It is common throughout Britain, including the Northern Isles and the Hebrides.[103]

ᔐ *Ivy*

A man from Lochnell, near Benderloch, Argyll, told me that during and after the First World War ivy leaves were

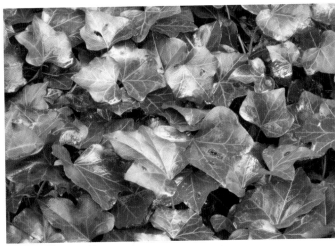

Opposite. Honeysuckle
Above. Ivy

used for healing wounds. Ivy (*Hedera helix*, in Gaelic 'Eidheann,' meaning possibly 'holding on') flowers in the late autumn, and is found throughout Britain in woodlands on trees, hedges and rocks, on all but very dry, very acid or very wet soils, up to 600 metres.[104]

Vegetables and kitchen cures

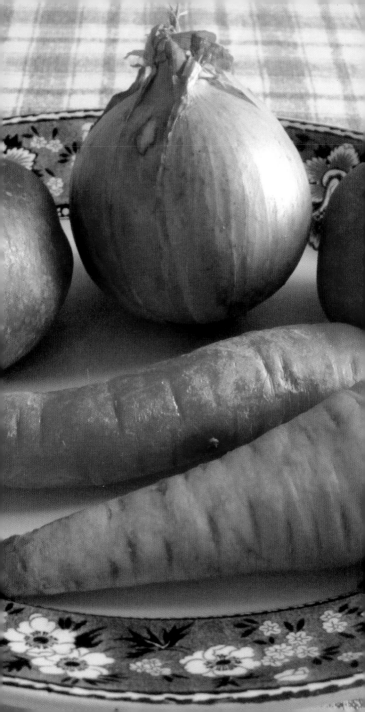

৪৯ *Eucalyptus Oil*

A woman from Quoyloo, Sandwick, Orkney, remembered that in the 1930s and '40s, when she lived on the Isle of Westray, a few drops of eucalyptus oil were dropped onto a handkerchief and breathed in for colds and sinus trouble. A native of Australia, the eucalyptus tree (*Eucalyptus globulus,* blue gum) was introduced in the 19th century to other parts of the world, including the Mediterranean, Africa and India, in malarial marshy areas, because the roots had a drying action on the soil. The medicinal oil is distilled from the fresh leaves of the tree.[105]

৪৯ *Linseed Meal*

When linseed, the seed of flax (*Linum usitatissimum*), is pressed for oil, there is a cake residue. This resulting oil-cake was used to fatten cattle, and linseed meal in former days used to be obtained by grinding up the oil-cake into powder.[106] In Brue on the Isle of Lewis, Mòr Macleod, who was the district nurse for the villages in that area from 1941, said that during the Second World War she called in to see a ten year old boy who had pneumonia. It was the most serious case she could remember. She wanted to make an oatmeal poultice (Oatmeal, p.101) for his chest and back, to help 'sweat out' the infection, but there wasn't any oatmeal left in the house. Everything was rationed at that time, and the family wouldn't be able to get any more oatmeal from Stornoway until their next ration cards came.

So, forced to improvise, Mòr asked whether they had any 'cattle cubes' (containing 'linseed meal and other things to feed the cattle in winter') on the croft. They did, so she mixed these up with some water in a pot over the fire, as for porridge, to make a hot poultice. This 'porridge' was placed between two layers of old sheeting and laid on the boy's back and chest. She spent all night long making poultices for the boy, changing them every twenty minutes, so that they were always hot. She also made him drink as much water as he could to encourage sweating. And the boy survived.

🙖 Mustard

A woman who grew up in Tenston, Sandwick, Orkney, said that when she was a child in the 1930s, if she had a 'bailin' (a festering boil), her mother (who was from the

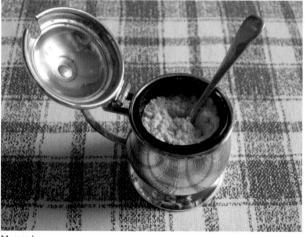

Mustard

Isle of Sanday) would take a slice of bread (Wheat, p.114), soak it in hot water, squeeze the bread out, and then put dry mustard (*Brassica nigra*) on it. This was then put over the boil and covered on top with muslin cloth as a poultice: 'it would draw the boil right out', but it would be very 'nippy'. She added that she was the eldest of nine children in the family; they had very little money, and no car. They couldn't afford to go to the doctor for ordinary ills, but if one of them did need the doctor, her father would have to get on his bicycle to fetch him. Black Mustard, cultivated in rich soils in Britain for its seed, is used both medicinally and as a condiment.[107]

Oatmeal

Oatmeal, the ground grain of oats (*Avena sativa*) often cultivated locally in Scotland, had many uses. A woman

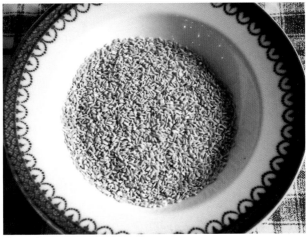

Oatmeal

from Uig, Skye, told me that her mother, who came from Lewis, used to make a refreshing, cooling drink from oatmeal water as follows: 'Steep medium oatmeal overnight in water. Discard oatmeal and drink the water.' The same woman told me that she gave her own children oatmeal jelly from the age of three months, as a weaning food. She made it by soaking medium oatmeal overnight in water. In the morning, the water was drained off into a saucepan, heated gently and stirred until it formed a jelly (the oatmeal was then cooked separately for porridge). In the days just after the Second World War, it was possible, she said, to buy packets of MOF (Midlothian Oat Flour – a powdered form of oatmeal jelly) from the meal shop.

An eighty year old man told me that his grandfather, a Cambridge-trained scientist living near Arisaig at the end of the 19th century, observed that the locals kept very well through the winter despite the lack of fresh fruit and vegetables; on further enquiry, he noted that they took a teaspoonful of fresh raw pinhead oatmeal, harvested locally, each morning on top of their cooked porridge.

A fisherman from Talmine, Sutherland, told me that for the older fishermen, who complained of a bad back after a cold night's fishing, a hot poultice of oatmeal was made and applied to the back, where it was left on overnight until the 'wee small hours'. He remembered his father and grandfather sailing the fishing smacks from Talmine to the big landing ports until the 1930s. A man from Easter Ross, who, as a child, had lived in Culrain, Sutherland, remembered that in the early 1930s his mother, who suffered from 'a bad chest', would have an oatmeal poultice applied to her chest, and was then wrapped up well. A similar poultice for a bad chest was made from thick porridge and put between sheets of brown paper (or strips of sheeting) before being placed on the chest and back, as I was told by several contributors from Quarff and Cunningsburgh, Shetland, who remember this from the late 1920s. Another man told me that, when he was a boy of seven in Altandubh, near Achiltibuie, Wester Ross, just before the First World War, his mother (who was herself born in 1870) would treat a bruise by making up oatmeal porridge, placing it warm on the bruise, wrapping it up with cloth, and leaving it on until the bruise eased.

Mòr Macleod in Brue, Lewis, remembered that before the Second World War, 'lots of people died of pneumonia in those days'; as a district nurse in that area from 1941, when no penicillin was available, she frequently used hot oatmeal poultices for serious chest infections. For a thumb infection, she said, a small oatmeal poultice would be placed over the boil, which brought it to a head; then it would be lanced with a pair of sharp scissors.

Hazel Gray in Camb, Mid Yell, Shetland, said that in the early 1960s, when she was a child playing outside at Aywick, East Yell, if she cut her finger or got a 'skelf' that went deep, her mother would put an oatmeal poultice on it, with a 'finger bag' over the top, to be left on overnight. In the morning, 'if the offending thing had not removed itself, a new poultice would be applied'. Similarly, a woman born in Gossabrough, East Yell, told me that her mother (born in Aywick in 1889) would use an oatmeal poultice for a 'baelin', that is 'anything gone

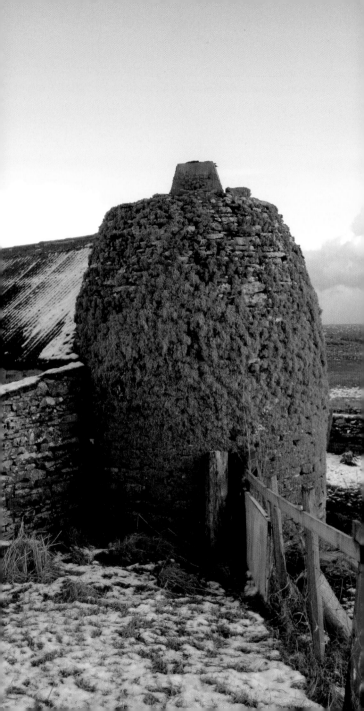

septic'. She remembers her mother using this on her in the 1930s.

Helen Jamieson, who was born in 1907 on a croft near Gossabrough, East Yell, told me that when she was little and had 'a bad chest', her aunts, who looked after her, made a very thick poultice from oatmeal and placed it between two layers of sheeting on her chest. They wrapped her up in bed and changed the poultice when it got cold. This happened before the First World War.

As an adult, she grew Shetland oats on the croft at Gossabrough. The threshed oats were dried in an old iron kettle over the fire, and stirred with a wooden spatula. When dry, they were ground in a hand mill. The meal was mixed with milk for 'burstin', used to make cakes (similar to oatcakes). In Skelberry, Dunrossness, Shetland, these cakes were known as 'burstin brunnies',

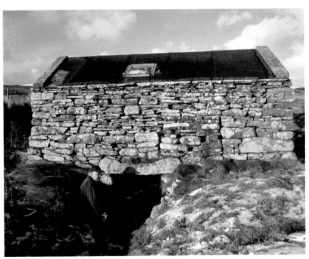

Opposite. Coarn kiln, Dunrossness, Shetland
Above. Bertie Johnson, watermill, Dunrossness

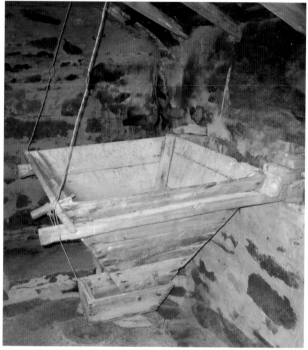

Grinding oats, watermill

a 'kind of bannack'. Near Skelberry there is a 'coarn' kiln, where the threshed grain is dried before grinding (the lichen-covered beehive shape, p.104).

Bertie Johnson grinds his own oats at a watermill (previous page) in Dunrossness, near his croft. The grindstone can get up to a speed of 60 rpm, with the water flowing through the wooden paddle wheel in the chamber below it. The meal emerges from a channel below the grindstone onto the floor.

It was the Romans who first introduced the culti-vated variety of oats to southern Britain.[108]

♊ *Oil of Cloves*

A woman from Sandwick, Orkney, told me that when they had toothache in the 1930s, her mother would put 'a few wee drops' of oil of cloves on the bad tooth 'and it was really good'. In those days in Sandwick, she said, there were no shops or chemists. Each day the horse-drawn vans would come over (and twice on Saturdays), and if they didn't have what you wanted that day you ordered what you needed from them. That's where they bought oil of cloves.

Cloves (*Eugenia caryophyllata*) are the undeveloped flowers of a small tropical evergreen tree from the Molucca Islands. The spice was first introduced into Europe around the 4th century, and the volatile medicinal oil is obtained from fresh cloves that are dark brown, fat, oily and aromatic.[109]

♊ *Olive Oil*

A woman from Dounby, Orkney, said that when she was a child in the late 1930s, if she had an earache, her mother would take one teaspoon filled with olive oil (from the Olive, *Olea europaea*), heat it over a match, then pour it into the sore ear and plug it with cotton wool. Similarly, a woman from Sandwick, Orkney, remembers that in the 1930s, for an earache, her mother would heat a knitting needle in hot water, dip it into the neck of the olive oil bottle, and then drop the (now hot) drops of oil into her sore ear; she then had to lie on her side to keep the oil in. For a sore throat, her mother would give her

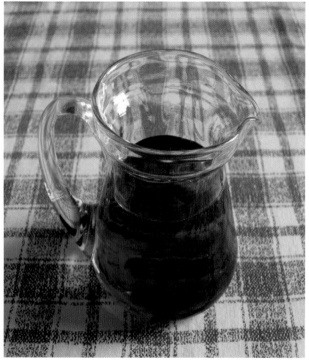

Olive oil

a teaspoon of olive oil with sugar. And for a chesty cough she would rub olive oil on her chest. In their house, olive oil was only ever used medicinally.

A native of Asia Minor, the olive tree is a small evergreen widely cultivated across the Mediterranean, especially in Italy and Spain; the oil is obtained from pressing the ripe fruits.[110]

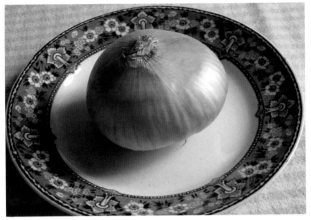

Onion

۶۵ Onion

Onion (*Allium cepa*), still widely cultivated in kitchen gardens and allotments, was a popular remedy in Scotland. A woman in Leith said that when she was a little girl in the 1920s and had a sore throat, her Caithness grandmother would chop up an onion, put it into a woollen sock, and wrap it around the child's neck.

A man from Quarff, Shetland, told me that as a child in 1927, when he had chest trouble his mother took an onion, pulled off the loose skin from it, and pushed it into the hot ashes of the fire. The onion was heated up, and then made into a poultice for the chest. A woman from Balmaqueen, Skye, said that for breast cancer a poultice of onion was used: 'The onion eats up the cancer.' A man from Skinnet, Talmine, in Sutherland remembered that when he was a child in the 1930s a poultice of onion was placed on a very sore joint. A man from Staffin, Skye, told me this story, which he had heard from people in the village who knew the man mentioned:

> In Staffin at the end of the First World War, the Spanish influenza came, brought by the soldiers from the trenches. The flu killed more people than had died in the war. There were three funerals a day in the village. People were so afraid of getting the flu that they stopped visiting each other; they closed their doors and windows. When someone died, the empty coffin was passed through the window of the house, the corpse was put into the coffin by those inside, and then the coffin was passed out again, the window shutting behind it. But one man was not afraid to visit the houses in the village, and he never got the flu. When it was all over, he was asked how he had survived. He answered that each morning he took an onion, cut it in half, and put one half under each oxter.[111] When he removed the onions at night, they had turned black. He did this each day until the flu was over.

A woman in Dounby, Orkney, told me that when she was a child, living on the Isle of Rousay, her mother (born in 1890) would treat an earache by taking half a fresh onion and squeezing the juice straight into the ear, and eventually the earache would get better. Another woman in Dounby told me that in the 1930s, when she lived on Rousay, her cousin used to hang half a raw onion from the roof inside to avoid a cold that might be going around the place. It was kept hanging there until the infection had passed. A third woman remembers that in Dounby in the 1940s her aunt would make up a cough mixture for them consisting of an onion, juiced and added to some honey and vinegar, which 'tasted terrible'.

Mòr Macleod of Brue told me that it was too wet to grow onions on crofts on the west side of Lewis, so they had to be bought from Stornoway. For a very sore throat (tonsillitis, she said it would be), they would parboil the bought onions, and put them in a cotton stocking and tie it round the neck.

ɣ Potato

The garden potato (*Solanum tuberosum*, Gaelic 'buntàta'[112]) provides a number of remedies. The potato was first introduced into Scotland as a garden plant in 1725, and by 1760 it was being grown in open fields.[113]

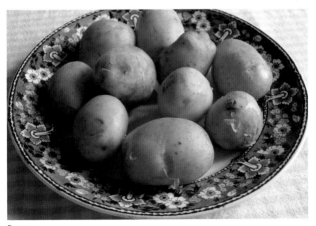

Potato

Morag Henriksen, who was brought up in Loch-carron, Wester Ross, remembers that her uncle believed that carrying a potato in his pocket would cure his rheumatism. As the potato wizened, 'it lost its power to keep the twinges at bay', so when it dried up he changed it for a fresh one. Her father tried it himself for a bit, 'but it never worked so well for him, maybe because he was sceptical'. Her mother, on the other hand, was 'openly contemptuous of such "old superstition"'.

A woman from Skye remembers that, for strains and sprains, her mother put 'grated raw potato between gauze' on the affected area, to help reduce the swelling and bruising. A woman from Achnahuaigh, Sutherland, said that before the Second World War her parents and grandparents in Talmine had used cooked potatoes as a poultice for a sore throat, and as a poultice on the chest for tuberculosis.

𝒫 Tobacco

A native plant of Virginia, tobacco (*Nicotiana tabacum*), in the same family as potato, was introduced into England in 1586, and has been cultivated locally in many parts of the world.[114] I collected these two stories within a day of each other, the first in Sutherland, the second in Easter Ross. Mary Beith in Sutherland related a story that she had been told by the late Mary Gunn Mackay (born in 1909), of Melness. When Mary Gunn was a little girl, around 1912 in Port Vasgo, she cut her palm badly, and it was bleeding. Someone set off in a horse and cart to fetch the doctor, who was more than ten miles away at

Tongue; but he wouldn't be able to get to her for several hours. Mary's mother took her to see Hector Pope at Talmine. Hector grew tobacco, for smoking purposes, down near the shore. Hector looked at Mary's hand, took a fresh leaf of tobacco, placed it on her bleeding palm, and folded her fingers over it. When the doctor arrived some time later, Mary's mother, rather shame-facedly, told him what she had done. The doctor asked to see the child's hand, then looked up at her mother and said that she couldn't have done anything better. The tobacco leaf had stopped the bleeding.

When I told this story the next day to another man in Easter Ross, he remembered a similar case. When he was a boy at Altandubh, Wester Ross, around 1914, his brother cut his arm very badly on the seashore. They were thirty-eight miles away from the nearest doctor. His father took out his pouch of Black XXX Twist tobacco, unrolled a leaf of it and carefully placed it over the wound. Then his mother bandaged it up. The tobacco stopped the bleeding and helped to heal the wound.

ɣ *Turnip*

Nicol Stove told me that in the 1930s in Sandwick, Shetland, 'neeps' (turnips, *Brassica rapa*),[115] grown on the croft, were boiled up with sugar: you took a spoonful of juice for a cold. Several people told me that snowball neeps, a small sweet white turnip, used to be eaten raw by children straight from the field near Gossabrough on Yell, as well as in Sandwick and Quarff on mainland Shetland.

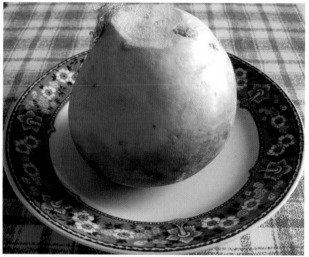

Turnip

❧ Wheat

In Aywick, East Yell, Shetland, a bread poultice (brown or white, home-made bread, from wheat, *Triticum aestivum*)[116] was used for surface cuts and small splinters, according to Hazel Gray of Camb, Mid Yell. To make the poultice, 'break up the bread in a cup with a little warm water, then mix, place over the splinter and bandage with gauze', with a 'finger bag' over the top of it. This was left on overnight. A man from Sandwick, Shetland, was given a bread poultice for an infected finger in the 1930s.

In Cunningsburgh, Shetland, in 1969, a bread poultice was used for a boil: bread, baking soda and hot water were mixed and spread on a muslin cloth, then folded over: 'you had to test it for temperature, so that it didn't burn you – but as hot as you could bear it'. This

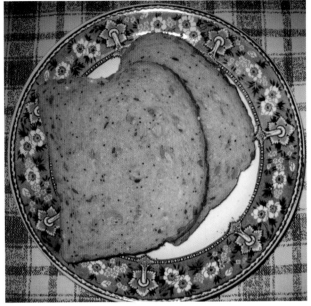

Wheat

was left on as long as necessary. This remedy originates with a woman who was born in 1913 in Quarff, Shetland, and was told to me by her daughter-in-law.

๕๐ Whisky

Whisky, made from malt produced from the steeping and drying of cultivated barley (*Hordeum distichon*[117]), features in several remedies from Sutherland. Mary Beith passed on to me a story told to her by Marion MacLeod, who was fourteen at the time of the incident, around 1910, in Skinnet, Melness. Marion was suffering badly from tonsillitis and had a quinsy[118] in her throat.

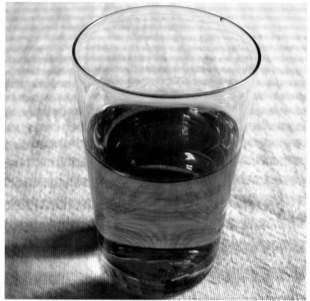

Whisky

An old woman visited her mother, and gave Marion the cure, which was to take a good half cup of whisky, and drink it neat, straight down. The cure worked so well that Marion was able to attend a wedding the very next day.

A man from Skinnet, Talmine, Sutherland, who had been a fisherman, remembered that when the older folks had been out all night on the fishing boats, and might have been feeling 'shivery' or feverish with a cold when they came in, were given a hot toddy (a good glass of whisky, and half again as much hot water, sweetened with sugar), which they drank and then went to bed to 'sweat it out'.

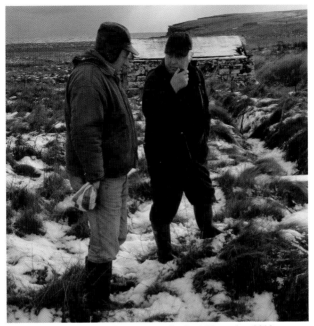

Crofters at a watermill in Dunrossness, Shetland, November 2010

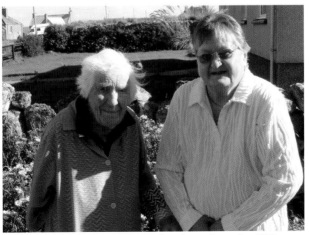

Mòr Macleod and Agnus Maclennan in Brue, Lewis, September 2010

✢ *Plant names and families*

Common	Scientific[119]	Family
Ash	*Fraxinus excelsior* L.	Oleaceae
Barley	*Hordeum distichon* L.[120]	Gramineae
Bay Willow	*Salix pentandra* L.	Salicaceae
Betony, Wood	*Stachys officinalis* (L.) Trevisan	Labiatae
Black Currant	*Ribes nigrum* L.	Grossulariaceae
Blaeberry	*Vaccinium myrtillus* L.	Ericaceae
Bog Bean	*Menyanthes trifoliata* L.	Menyanthaceae
Bog Cotton	*Eriophorum angustifolium* L.	Cyperaceae
Bog Myrtle	*Myrica gale* L.	Myricaceae
Bramble	*Rubus fruticosus* L. agg.	Rosaceae
Broad Bent, Marram	*Ammophila arenaria* (L.) Link	Gramineae
Butterwort	*Pinguicula vulgaris* L.	Lentibulariaceae
Carrageen	*Chondrus crispus* Stackh.[121]	Gigartinaceae
Chickweed	*Stellaria media* L.	Caryophyllaceae
Clove	*Eugenia caryophyllata* Thumb.	Myrtaceae
Crottal	*Parmelia* spp.[122]	Parmeliaceae
Crowberry	*Empetrum nigrum* L.	Empetraceae
Dandelion	*Taraxacum officinale* (*Vulgaria* Dahlst.)	Compositae
Docken		
(Broad-leaved)	*Rumex obtusifolius* L.	Polygonaceae
(Curled)	*Rumex crispus* L.	Polygonaceae
(Northern)	*Rumex longifolius* D.C.	Polygonaceae
Dulse	*Palmaria palmata* (L.) Weber & Mohr[123]	Palmariaceae
Eucalyptus	*Eucalyptus globulus* Labill.[124]	Myrtaceae
Eyebright	*Euphrasia arctica* Lange ex. Rostrup[125]	Orobanchaceae
Field Scabious	*Knautia arvensis* (L.) Coulter	Dipsacaceae
Foxglove	*Digitalis purpurea* L.	Plantaginaceae
Fucus, Channelled	*Pelvetia canaliculata* (L.) Dcne. & Thur.[126]	Fucaceae
Gooseberry	*Ribes uva-crispa* L.	Grossulariaceae
Haws (Hawthorn)	*Crataegus monogyna* Jacq.	Rosaceae
Heather	*Calluna vulgaris* (L.) Hull	Ericaceae

Common	Scientific	Family
Hips		
(Dog Rose)	*Rosa canina* L.	Rosaceae
(Northern Dog Rose)	*Rosa caesia* Sm.	Rosaceae
Honeysuckle	*Lonicera periclymenum* L.	Caprifoliaceae
Houseleek	*Sempervivum tectorum* L.	Crassulaceae
Ivy	*Hedera helix* L.	Araliaceae
Linseed	*Linum usitatissimum* L.	Linaceae
Meadowsweet	*Filipendula ulmaria* (L.) Maxim	Rosaceae
Milkwort	*Polygala serpyllifolia* J.A.C. Hose	Polygalaceae
Mustard	*Brassica nigra* (L.) Koch	Cruciferae
Nettle (Stinging)	*Urtica dioica* L.	Urticaceae
Oats (and Chaff)	*Avena sativa* L.[127]	Gramineae
Olive	*Olea europaea* L.[128]	Oleaceae
Onion	*Allium cepa* L.[129]	Amaryllidaceae
Pignut	*Conopodium majus* (Gouan) Loret	Umbelliferae
Potato	*Solanum tuberosum* L.[130]	Solanaceae
Primrose	*Primula vulgaris* Hudson	Primulaceae
Rat-tail Plantain	*Plantago major* L.	Plantaginaceae
Ribwort	*Plantago lanceolata* L.	Plantaginaceae
Roseroot	*Sedum rosea* (L). Scop.	Crassulaceae
St John's Wort, Common	*Hypericum perforatum* L.	Hypericaceae
St John's Wort, Slender	*Hypericum pulchrum* L.	Hypericaceae
Silverweed	*Potentilla anserina* L.	Rosaceae
Sorrel (Sooracks)	*Rumex acetosa* L.	Polygonaceae
Sphagnum (and Peat)	*Sphagnum* spp.[131]	Sphagnaceae
Thistle, Melancholy	*Cirsium helenioides* (L.) Hill	Compositae
Tobacco	*Nicotiana tabacum* L.[132]	Solanaceae
Tormentil	*Potentilla erecta* (L.) Räuschel	Rosaceae
Turnip (Neeps)	*Brassica rapa* L.	Cruciferae
Watercress	*Nasturtium officinale* R. Br.	Cruciferae
Wheat	*Triticum aestivum* L.[133]	Gramineae
Whisky (from Barley)	*Hordeum distichon* L.[134]	Gramineae
Yarrow	*Achillea millefolium* L.	Compositae
Yellow Rattle	*Rhinanthus minor* L.	Orobanchaceae

✌ *Notes*

1 Milliken, W. and Bridgewater, S., *Flora Celtica,* pp. 16–20, passim.
2 John MacInnes, in preface to Carmichael, A., *Carmina Gadelica*, p. 8.
3 Ibid., p. 23.
4 Ibid., pp. 152–6, passim; Dwelly, E., *Illustrated Gaelic-English Dictionary* (referred to as 'Dwelly') defines Mòthan as 'Bog Violet', *Pinguicula vulgaris* (Butterwort and Milkwort p.4). See also Scott, M., *Scottish Wild Flowers*, p. 203.
5 *Healing Threads: Traditional Medicines of the Highlands and Islands*.
6 Milliken and Bridgewater, *Flora Celtica*, p. 23.
7 Clapham, A.R., Tutin, T.G. and Warburg, E.F., *Excursion Flora of the British Isles*, p. 288; Blamey, M., Fitter, R. and Fitter, A., *Wild Flowers of Britain & Ireland*, p. 218.
8 Vice county recorder for the Botanical Society of the British Isles for the Isle of Raasay, and for Portree on the Isle of Skye.
9 Scott, *Scottish Wild Flowers*, p. 191.
10 Ibid., p. 203.
11 Ibid., p. 203; Blamey *et al*, *Wild Flowers*, p. 250; Clapham *et al*, *Excursion Flora*, p. 277.
12 Scott, *Scottish Wild Flowers*, p. 191; Blamey *et al*, *Wild Flowers*, p. 170; Clapham *et al*, *Excursion Flora*, p. 74.
13 Shetland dialect for 'devil the thing', i.e. nothing.
14 Scott, W. and Palmer, R., *The Flowering Plants and Ferns of the Shetland Islands*, p. 257; for details of subspecies, see pp. 257–64.
15 *Euphrasia arctica* Lange ex. Rostrup, subspecies *arctica*, is found only in Orkney, Shetland and Faeroe, Ibid., p. 257; Blamey *et al*, *Wild Flowers*, p. 236, indicate that *E. arctica* is the most common species found in Scotland; see also Clapham *et al*, *Excursion Flora*, p. 272.
16 Scott, *Scottish Wild Flowers*, p. 82.
17 Dwelly has 'Gille guirmen', as does Scott, *Scottish Wild Flowers*, p. 89.
18 Scott, *Scottish Wild Flowers*, p. 89; Blamey *et al*, *Wild Flowers*, pp. 262–3; Clapham *et al*, *Excursion Flora*, p. 311.
19 I photographed this eyebright (possibly *Euphrasia arctica*) at Skipi Geo, Birsay, Orkney, in August 2010.
20 According to Scott, another Gaelic name is 'Lus nam Ban-Sìdh', 'Fairy Women's plant' (*Scottish Wild Flowers*, p. 38).
21 Scott, *Scottish Wild Flowers*, p. 38; Blamey *et al*, *Wild Flowers*, p. 232; Clapham *et al*, *Excursion Flora*, p. 266.
22 Scott, *Scottish Wild Flowers*, p. 159.
23 Ibid., p. 159; Blamey *et al*, *Wild Flowers*, p. 128; Clapham *et al*, *Excursion Flora*, p. 139.

24 Shetland dialect for 'rubbish', i.e. no good.

25 'Takuusiemen Kaura Havre', according to the label on a sack of seed.

26 Scott, *Scottish Wild Flowers*, p. 138.

27 Dwelly.

28 Scott, *Scottish Wild Flowers*, p. 138; Blamey *et al*, *Wild Flowers*,
    p. 186; Clapham *et al*, *Excursion Flora*, p. 192.

29 Scott, *Scottish Wild Flowers*, p. 74.

30 Also called 'Barks', both local Shetland names for tormentil, according to Jill.

31 Scott, *Scottish Wild Flowers*, p. 74; Blamey *et al*, *Wild Flowers*,
    p. 130; Clapham *et al*, *Excursion Flora*, pp. 144–5.

32 Scott, *Scottish Wild Flowers*, p. 192.

33 Beith, *Healing Threads*, p. 238.

34 Scott, *Scottish Wild Flowers*, p. 192.

35 Ibid., p. 192; Blamey *et al*, *Wild Flowers*, p. 72; Clapham *et al*, *Excursion Flora*,
    p. 76.

36 Scott, *Scottish Wild Flowers*, p. 90.

37 Ibid., p. 90; Blamey *et al*, *Wild Flowers*, p. 268; Clapham *et al*, *Excursion
    Flora*, p. 332.

38 Hughes, G., Davies, N., and Moncrieff H., *Living Shetland Biodiversity
    Action Plan*, p. 11.

39 Johnston, J.L., *A Naturalist's Shetland*, p. 398; see also Scott and Palmer,
    Flowering Plants, p. 267; Clapham *et al*, *Excursion Flora*, p. 271, Blamey *et al*,
    Wild Flowers, p. 234, Scott, *Scottish Wild Flowers*, p. 82.

40 Dwelly. Scott, *Scottish Wild Flowers*, p. 51, equates Fliodh with 'excrescence'.

41 Ibid., p. 51; Blamey *et al*, *Wild Flowers*, p. 50; Clapham *et al*, *Excursion Flora*,
    p. 89.

42 Scott, *Scottish Wild Flowers*, p. 92.

43 Ibid., p. 92; Blamey *et al*, *Wild Flowers*, p. 294; Clapham *et al*, *Excursion
    Flora*, p. 374.

44 Probably *Rumex obtusifolius* L., Broad-leaved dock, which often hybridises
    with *R. crispus* L., Curled dock; see Clapham *et al*, *Excursion Flora*, pp. 210–11.

45 *Rumex acetosa*, Scott, *Scottish Wild Flowers*, p. 77

46 Ibid., pp. 34–5.

47 Blamey *et al*, *Wild Flowers*, pp. 60–4; Clapham *et al*, *Excursion Flora*, pp.
    208–11. Scott and Palmer, *Flowering Plants*, pp. 116–17, note that in Shetland,
    the Northern Dock (*R. longifolius*) is the most common, while Broad Dock
    has colonised areas near crofts.

48 Scott, *Scottish Wild Flowers*, p. 29; Blamey *et al*, *Wild Flowers*,
    p. 124; Clapham *et al*, *Excursion Flora*, p. 154.

49 Blamey *et al*, *Wild Flowers*, p. 390; Clapham *et al*, *Excursion Flora*, p. 158.

50 Scott, *Scottish Wild Flowers*, p. 53.

51 Ibid., p. 53; Blamey *et al*, *Wild Flowers*, p. 36; Clapham *et al*, *Excursion Flora*,
    p. 212.

52 Scott, *Scottish Wild Flowers*, p. 87.

53 Jill Blackadder, of Scalloway, Shetland, told me that she had been told this
    by a number of Shetlanders over the past twenty years.

54 Scott, *Scottish Wild Flowers*, p. 87; Blamey *et al*, *Wild Flowers*,
    p. 248; Clapham *et al*, *Excursion Flora*, pp. 294–5.

55 Clapham *et al*, *Excursion Flora*, p. 340; Scott, *Scottish Wild Flowers*, p. 91, has
    synonym *C. heterophyllum*.

56 Blamey *et al*, *Wild Flowers*, p. 290; Clapham *et al*, *Excursion Flora*, p. 341.

57 Scott, *Scottish Wild Flowers*, p. 198.

58 In Dwelly, 'curach' means fen or bog, but 'mheig' is obscure.

59   Scott, *Scottish Wild Flowers*, p. 198; Blamey *et al*, *Wild Flowers*, p. 106; Clapham *et al*, *Excursion Flora*, pp. 233–4.

60   'Smeur' means berry in Scott, *Scottish Wild Flowers*, p. 28.

61   Ibid., p. 28; Blamey *et al*, *Wild Flowers*, p. 126; Clapham *et al*, *Excursion Flora*, p. 142.

62   In Dwelly, 'crotal' refers to *Parmelia saxatilis* and *P. omphalodes*, the stone- or heath-parmelia.

63   Clapham *et al*, *Excursion Flora*, p. 236; Scott, *Scottish Wild Flowers*, p. 201; Blamey *et al*, *Wild Flowers*, p.102.

64   Scott, *Scottish Wild Flowers*, p. 200.

65   Ibid., p. 200; Blamey *et al*, *Wild Flowers*, p. 104; Clapham *et al*, *Excursion Flora*, pp. 231–2.

66   Scott, *Scottish Wild Flowers*, p. 139; Dwelly has 'Sòbhrag'.

67   Literally 'bad blood', according to Agnus, meaning anaemia or an infection in the blood.

68   Scott, *Scottish Wild Flowers*, p. 139; Blamey *et al*, *Wild Flowers*, p. 110; Clapham *et al*, *Excursion Flora*, p. 240.

69   According to Clapham *et al*, *Excursion Flora*, p. 162, synonymous with *Rhodiola rosea*.

70   Scott, *Scottish Wild Flowers*, p. 160.

71   Ibid., p. 106; see also Dwelly, who calls it Roseroot, *Sedum rhodiola*, synonymous with *S. rosea*.

72   Clapham *et al*, *Excursion Flora*, p. 162.

73   Winston, D. and Maimes, S., *Adaptogens*, p. 192.

74   Grieve, M., *A Modern Herbal*, pp. 422–3.

75   According to Mary Beith.

76   Scott, *Scottish Wild Flowers*, p. 212; Blamey *et al*, *Wild Flowers*, p. 214; Clapham *et al*, *Excursion Flora*, p. 248.

77   Clapham *et al*, *Excursion Flora*, p. 427; Blamey *et al*, *Wild Flowers*, pp. 434–5; Scott, *Scottish Wild Flowers*, p. 210.

78   Scott, *Scottish Wild Flowers*, p. 196.

79   Ibid., p. 196; Blamey *et al*, *Wild Flowers*, p. 362; Clapham *et al*, *Excursion Flora*, p. 215.

80   According to Dr David Chamberlain of the Royal Botanic Garden, Edinburgh.

81   Beith, *Healing Threads*, p. 243.

82   According to Dr David Chamberlain of the Royal Botanic Garden, Edinburgh.

83   Grieve, *A Modern Herbal*, pp. 552–3.

84   Clapham *et al*, *Excursion Flora*, p. 64.

85   Scott, *Scottish Wild Flowers*, p. 156, has Gaelic 'Biolair Uisge'.

86   According to Kathryn Watt, researcher at the University of Edinburgh.

87   Blamey *et al*, *Wild Flowers*, p. 90; Clapham *et al*, *Excursion Flora*, p. 64.

88   Clapham *et al*, *Excursion Flora*, p. 467; Blamey *et al*, *Wild Flowers*, pp. 420–1.

89   Dwelly has 'an Cairgein', Irish moss, from the Irish 'Carragheen', diminutive of 'carraig', meaning rock or cliff; 'careagan' is the local name in Staffin.

90   Grieve, *A Modern Herbal*, p. 552.

91   Dwelly.

92   Dwelly has *Fucus canaliculatus*, which is synonymous with *Pelvetia canaliculata*.

93   Shetland name for seaweed.

94   Clapham *et al*, *Excursion Flora*, p. 243.

95   Dwelly.

96   Beith, *Healing Threads*, p. 203.

97 Blamey *et al*, *Wild Flowers*, p. 388; Clapham *et al*, *Excursion Flora*, p. 243.

98 Clapham *et al*, *Excursion Flora*, p. 226.

99 Ibid., p. 226; Blamey *et al*, *Wild Flowers*, p. 378.

100 Clapham *et al*, *Excursion Flora*, p. 169; Blamey *et al*, *Wild Flowers*, p. 392; Grieve, *A Modern Herbal*, pp. 243–4.

101 Clapham *et al*, *Excursion Flora*, p. 169; Blamey *et al*, *Wild Flowers*, p. 392.

102 Beith, *Healing Threads*, p. 223; Scott, *Scottish Wild Flowers*, p. 145.

103 Scott, *Scottish Wild Flowers*, p. 145; Blamey *et al*, *Wild Flowers*, p. 258; Clapham *et al*, *Excursion Flora*, p. 307.

104 Scott, *Scottish Wild Flowers*, p. 137; Blamey *et al*, *Wild Flowers*, p. 396; Clapham *et al*, *Excursion Flora*, p. 186.

105 Grieve, *A Modern Herbal*, pp. 287–9.

106 Ibid., p. 319.

107 Ibid., pp. 568–9.

108 Beith, Healing Threads, p. 33.

109 Grieve, *A Modern Herbal*, p. 208.

110 Ibid., pp. 598–9.

111 Armpit.

112 Dwelly.

113 Grieve, *A Modern Herbal*, p. 654.

114 Ibid., p. 817.

115 Pictured, the yellow-fleshed Swedish turnip, *B. napus* ssp. napobrassica (L.); *B. rapa* L. ssp. rapa is the cultivated white turnip, according to Clapham *et al*, *Excursion Flora*, pp. 48–9. In Scotland, 'neeps' may refer to either.

116 Blamey *et al*, *Wild Flowers*, p. 422.

117 Grieve, *A Modern Herbal*, pp. 84–5.

118 A pus-filled infection around the tonsils.

119 Clapham *et al*, *Excursion Flora*, is the source of all the scientific names and family classifications, unless otherwise indicated; however, some family classifications have changed in the past thirty years since Clapham came out, so where this is the case (foxglove, eyebright, yellow rattle) I have followed Stevens, P.F., Angiosperm Phylogeny Website. Where a family has two names (e.g. Cruciferae vs. Brassicaceae), I have followed Clapham *et al*.

120 Grieve, *A Modern Herbal*, p. 84.

121 Ibid., p. 552; Guiry, M.D. and Guiry, W.,'*Chondrus elatus* Holmes'.

122 Dwelly indicates *Parmelia saxatilis* and *P. omphalodes*. See note 62.

123 Guiry, M.D., '*Palmaria palmata* (Linnaeus) Weber & Mohr'.

124 Polunin, O. and Huxley, A., *Flowers of the Mediterranean,* p. 134.

125 Scott and Palmer, *Flowering Plants*, p. 257; according to Clapham *et al*, the species included under *Euphrasia officinalis* L., *sensu lato*, are extremely variable, frequently hybridise, and are difficult to determine (see *Excursion Flora*, p. 272).

126 Grieve, *A Modern Herbal,* p. 114; Guiry, M.D., '*Pelvetia canaliculata* (Linnaeus) Decaisne & Thuret'.

127 Grieve, *A Modern Herbal*, p. 597.

128 Polunin and Huxley, *Flowers*, p. 145.

129 Grieve, *A Modern Herbal*, p. 599.

130 Ibid., p. 654.

131 According to Dr David Chamberlain, there are 35 species of sphagnum in Britain, including *S. palustre* (synonym *S. cymbifolium*).

132 Grieve, *A Modern Herbal*, p. 817.

133 See Blamey *et al*, *Wild Flowers*, p. 422; USDA, '*Triticum aestivum* L.'.

134 Grieve, *A Modern Herbal*, p. 84.

124

℀ *Bibliography*

Beith, M., *Healing Threads: Traditional Medicines of the Highlands and Islands* (Edinburgh, Polygon, 1995)

Blamey, M., Fitter, R. and Fitter, A., *Wild Flowers of Britain & Ireland* (London, A. & C. Black, 2003)

Carmichael, A., *Carmina Gadelica* (Edinburgh, Floris, 1992)

Clapham, A.R., Tutin, T.G. and Warburg, E.F., *Excursion Flora of the British Isles* 3rd edn (Cambridge University Press, 1981)

Dwelly, E., *Illustrated Gaelic-English Dictionary* (Edinburgh, Birlinn, 2001)

Grieve, M., *A Modern Herbal* (New York, Dover, 1971)

Guiry, M.D., '*Palmaria palmata* (Linnaeus) Weber & Mohr' (Galway, Martin Ryan Institute, 2010) in algaeBASE (http://www.algaebase.org/search/species/detail/?species_id=1), accessed 18.8.10 at 14:00

Guiry, M.D., '*Pelvetia canaliculata* (Linnaeus) Decaisne & Thuret' (Galway, Martin Ryan Institute, 2008) in algaeBASE (http://www.algaebase.org/search/species/detail/?species_id=88), accessed 18.8.10 at 14:00

Guiry, M.D. and Guiry, W.,'*Chondrus elatus* Holmes' (Galway, Martin Ryan Institute, 2009) in algaeBASE (http://www.algaebase.org/search/species/detail/? species_id=3488), accessed 18.8.10 at 14:00

Hughes, G., Davies, N. and Moncrieff, H., *Living Shetland Biodiversity Action Plan* (Lerwick, Shetland Islands Council, 2004), p. 11 (http://www.shetland.gov.uk/conservation/documents/Roadsides.pdf), accessed 24.11.10 at 10:30

Johnston, J.L., *A Naturalist's Shetland* (London, T. & A.D. Poyser, 1999)

Milliken, W. and Bridgewater, S., *Flora Celtica* (Edinburgh, Birlinn, 2004)

Polunin, O. and Huxley, A., *Flowers of the Mediterranean* (London, Chatto & Windus, 1987)

Scott, M., *Scottish Wild Flowers* (Glasgow, Collins, 2000)

Scott, W. and Palmer, R., *The Flowering Plants and Ferns of the Shetland Islands* (Lerwick, Shetland Times, 1987)

Stevens, P.F., Angiosperm Phylogeny Website (St Louis, Missouri Botanical Garden, 2001 onwards {last updated 11.12.10}) (http://www.mobot.org/ MOBOT/research/APweb/) of which: 'OROBANCHACEAE Ventenat' http://www.mobot.org/mobot/research/apweb/generaorobanchaceaegen. html (accessed 16.12.10 at 10:40)
'PLANTAGINACEAE Jussieu' http://www.mobot.org/mobot/ research/apweb/genera/plantaginaceaegen.html (accessed 16.12.10 at 10:40)

USDA, '*Triticum aestivum* L.' in USDA Natural Resources Conservation Service
    (Washington, United States Department of Agriculture, 2010)
    (http://plants.usda.gov/java/profile?symbol=TRAE) accessed 6.12.10 at 14:30
Winston, D. and Maimes, S., *Adaptogens* (Rochester, Healing Arts Press, 2007)

❧ *Index*